Published by OnlineMedEd, www.onlinemeded.org
Authored by Dustyn Williams
Produced by Staci Weber

Printed in the United States of America

Congrats on making it through the first half of Basic Sciences. You're well on your way, but fair warning: it only gets harder from here on out. The foundation you build here in Basic Sciences will matter for the rest of your med school years (and beyond when you're practicing). Do yourself a favor, and make it a solid one.

Fortunately, you've found OnlineMedEd. I co-founded this company because I believe there's a better way to impart medical knowledge so that students actually understand and retain it. This book is a part of that mission.

This book:

- **IS** a companion to OnlineMedEd's free Basic Sciences lesson videos and a great place to take notes and reference our final whiteboards.

- **IS NOT** an excuse to skip the lessons or avoid writing your own notes.

In fact, I advocated against this book because I didn't want it used as a shortcut. **Skipping steps will compromise your learning.** Don't do it.

After I saw how much time, money, and energy you guys were putting into printing your own versions of my whiteboards, often in poor quality formats, I relented.

This book was born from OnlineMedEd's two guiding principles:

1. **Medical knowledge belongs to no one**, and so it is accessible to everyone. This is why the videos these whiteboards accompany are free and always will be.

2. **OnlineMedEd's PACE learning methodology** — reading the notes (and taking your own), watching the video (and taking more notes), doing the challenge questions (and... wait for it... taking more notes), and enforcing it all through repetition — works.

This book is a part of PACE, NOT a replacement for it. Purposeful engagement of the content in multiple modalities is the path to success. This is just one of those modalities.

I designed the lessons to flow a certain way. The positioning on the board, the order in which the material is presented, the colors used, and even the cadences of speech are not accidental. They're all purposefully designed to help you understand what you need to understand when you need to understand it.

You got this,

Dustyn Williams, MD

Table of Contents

NEUROSCIENCE

REPRODUCTION

Introduction to the Cardiac Module

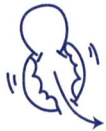

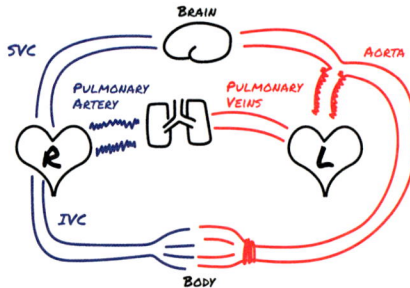

I: HEMODYNAMICS (8)
BLOOD VESSELS
BLOOD PRESSURE
SHOCK

$$MAP = CO \times SVR$$
$$HR \times SV$$
$$CONT \times PL$$

II: S+F (8)
ANATOMY / HISTOLOGY
INFLAMED
HEART AS A PUMP
VENTRICULAR MYOCYTE
HEART FAILURE
CARDIOMYOPATHY

III: PLUMBING (5)
EMBRYOGENESIS OF ♡
CONGENITAL
CARDIAC CYCLE
VALVES

IV: ELECTRICITY (5)
CONDUCTION ↔ CORONARY
ARRHYTHMIA
ECG, 12-LEAD
PACEMAKER MYOCYTE

V: CAD (6)
ATHEROSCLEROSIS
CHRONIC ISCHEMIC ♡
ACUTE CORONARY SYNDROME

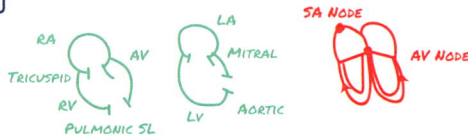

Arteries and Veins

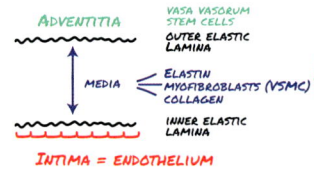

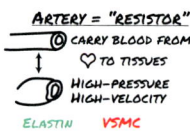

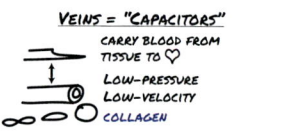

INTIMA = ENDOTHELIUM

LARGE ARTERIES = ELASTIC
AD: LOTS, VASA VASORUM
MED: ELASTIN (VSMC, COLLAGEN)
INT: LUMEN : MEDIA
     12 MM   2 M

MEDIUM ARTERIES = CONDUITS
AD: ALMOST NONE
MED: VSMC (ELASTIN, COLLAGEN)
INT: LUMEN : MEDIA
     2 MM   1 MM

ARTERIOLES
AD: ∅
MED: VSMC
INT: LUMEN : MEDIA
     15 MM   20 MM

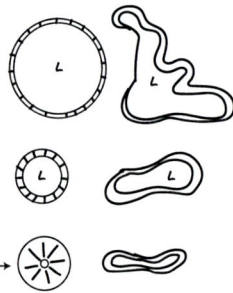

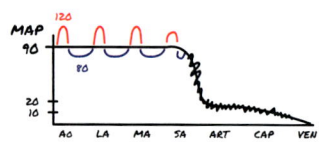

ARTERY = "RESISTOR"
CARRY BLOOD FROM
♡ TO TISSUES
HIGH-PRESSURE
HIGH-VELOCITY
ELASTIN   VSMC

VEINS = "CAPACITORS"
CARRY BLOOD FROM
TISSUE TO ♡
LOW-PRESSURE
LOW-VELOCITY
COLLAGEN

RESISTANCE
VASOCONSTRICTION

FLOW

$$RESISTANCE \propto \frac{1}{R^4}$$

$$RESISTANCE \propto \frac{1}{FLOW}$$

VASODILATION

NOTES

Capillaries

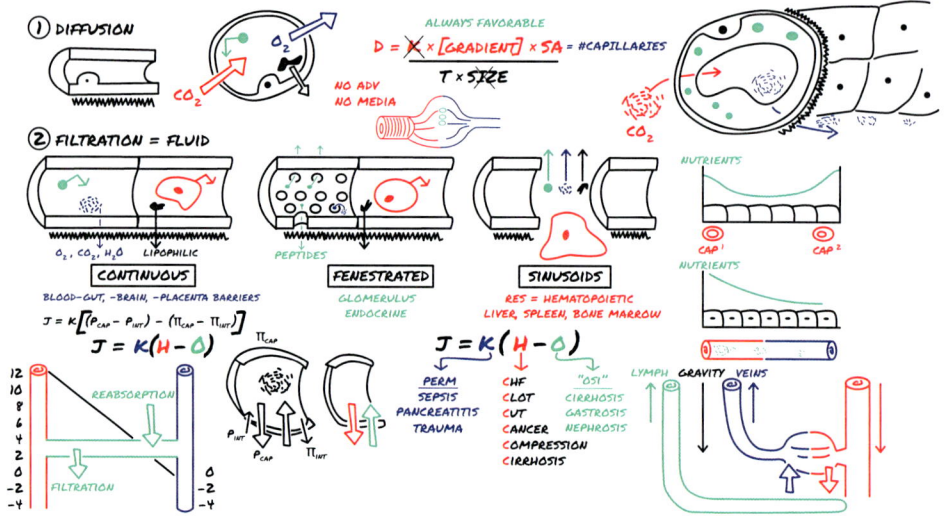

Aorta

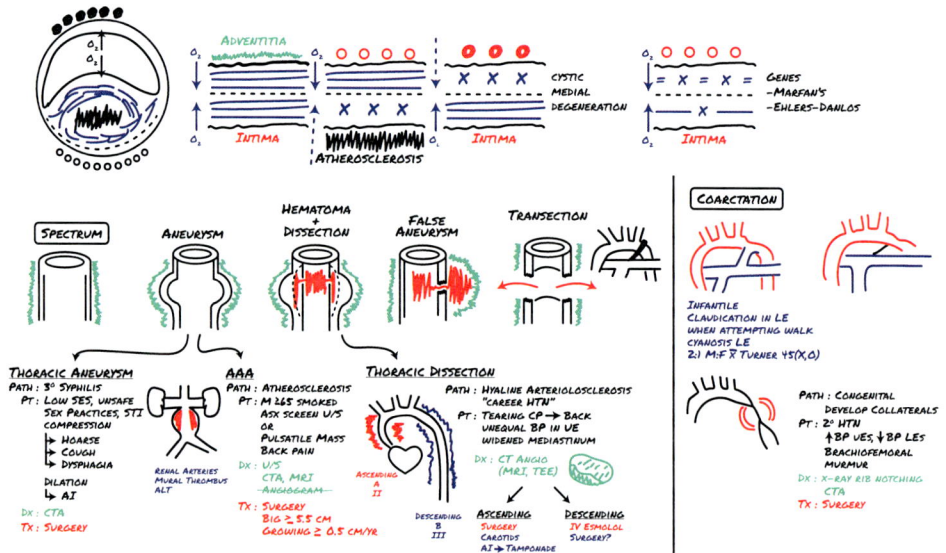

NOTES

Blood Pressure Regulation

SYSTEMIC

$$MAP = CO \times SVR$$

ARTERIOLAR TONE
α_1 - SNS
AT 1 - ANG-2

HEART — β_1, SNS

$$HR \times SV$$

$$CONT \times PL$$

VOLUME, Na⁺
ALDOSTERONE

RAAS (HORMONAL)

CHANGES MIN-HRS (ANG-2)
HRS-DAYS (ALDO)

AT 1

RENIN
OFF — ANG-2
ON
ALDO

BARORECEPTOR REFLEX (AUTONOMICS)

CHANGES IN SECONDS (NOREPI)
IN MINUTES (EPI)

NTS, MEDULLA
CN 9
CAROTID BODIES

SNS   PNS
CN 10   CN 10
AORTIC BODIES

α_1
β_2 M_2 β_1

$\alpha_1 = \uparrow SVR$
$\beta_2 = \uparrow HR$
$\beta_1 = \uparrow CONT$
$M_2 = \downarrow HR$

$\uparrow MAP = \uparrow STRETCH = \uparrow RATE OF$
FIRING OF BODIES

SNS
$\downarrow HR$
$\downarrow CONT$
$\downarrow SVR$
PNS

$\uparrow RATE IF$
FIRING OF NTS

CPP (SPECIAL)

$$CPP = MAP - ICP$$

β_1 α_1
$\uparrow HR \uparrow SVR$
$\uparrow CONT$

$M_2 = \downarrow HR$

$\uparrow MAP$
$\Downarrow HR$
CUSHING'S REFLEX

REGIONAL

WHEN STRETCHED, FIGHT BACK

Ca^{2+} Ca^{2+}

AUTOREGULATION

MYOGENIC RESPONSE

METABOLIC DEMAND (HYPEREMIA)

MORE FLOW
MORE NUTRIENTS   — $\uparrow CO_2$
— ADENOSINE   — $\downarrow O_2$
— LACTATE   — $\downarrow PH$
— NITRIC OXIDE

PULMONIC CIRCULATION

$\downarrow O_2$

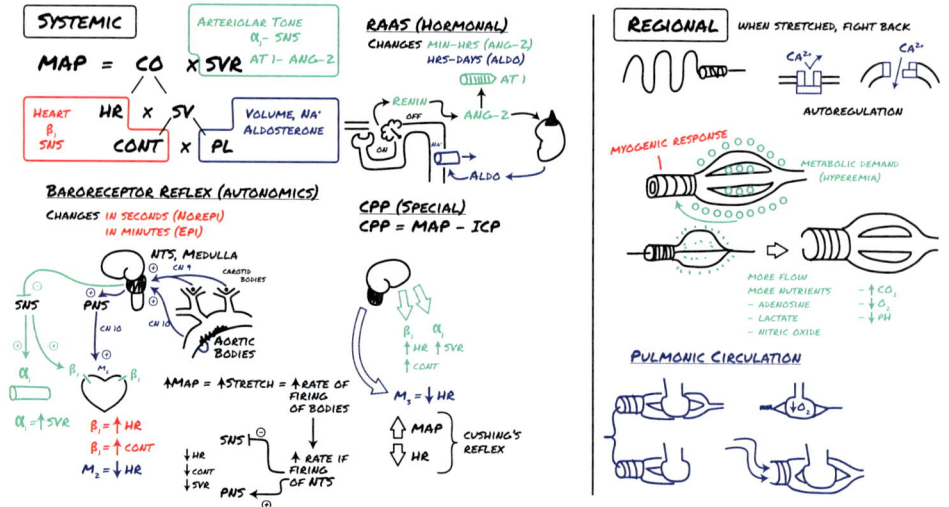

Essential Hypertension

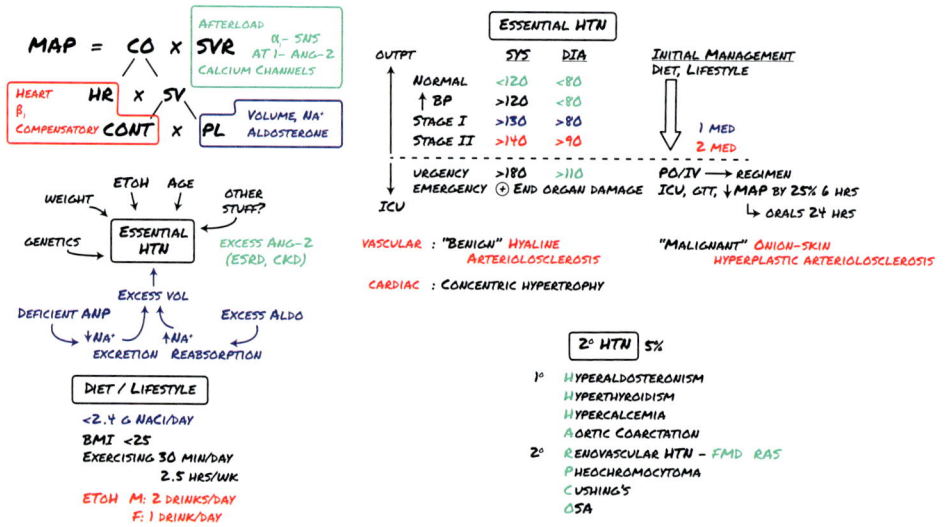

$$MAP = CO \times SVR$$

AFTERLOAD
α_1 - SNS
AT 1 - ANG-2
CALCIUM CHANNELS

HEART — β_1

$$HR \times SV$$

COMPENSATORY CONT $\times PL$

VOLUME, Na⁺
ALDOSTERONE

WEIGHT   ETOH   AGE   OTHER STUFF?

GENETICS → ESSENTIAL HTN → EXCESS ANG-2 (ESRD, CKD)

EXCESS VOL

DEFICIENT ANP   EXCESS ALDO
$\downarrow Na^+$ $\uparrow Na^+$
EXCRETION   REABSORPTION

DIET / LIFESTYLE

<2.4 G NaCl/DAY
BMI <25
EXERCISING 30 MIN/DAY
             2.5 HRS/WK
ETOH M: 2 DRINKS/DAY
      F: 1 DRINK/DAY

ESSENTIAL HTN	SYS	DIA
OUTPT NORMAL	<120	<80
↑ BP	>120	<80
STAGE I	>130	>80
STAGE II	>140	>90
URGENCY	>180	>110
EMERGENCY ⊕ END ORGAN DAMAGE		

INITIAL MANAGEMENT
DIET, LIFESTYLE

1 MED
2 MED

PO/IV → REGIMEN
ICU, GTT, $\downarrow$ MAP BY 25% 6 HRS
→ ORALS 24 HRS

VASCULAR : "BENIGN" HYALINE ARTERIOLOSCLEROSIS

CARDIAC : CONCENTRIC HYPERTROPHY

"MALIGNANT" ONION-SKIN HYPERPLASTIC ARTERIOLOSCLEROSIS

2° HTN 5%

1° HYPERALDOSTERONISM
   HYPERTHYROIDISM
   HYPERCALCEMIA
   AORTIC COARCTATION
2° RENOVASCULAR HTN – FMD RAS
   PHEOCHROMOCYTOMA
   CUSHING'S
   OSA

Hypertension Pharmacology

α₂-AGONISTS
1. CLONIDINE
   * REBOUND HTN *
2. α-METHYL-DOPA
   * DRUG-INDUCED LUPUS *

NOT ANTI HYPERTENSIVES
1. NDHP-CCB = RATE CONTROLS
   VERAPAMIL + DILTIAZEM
2. α₁ ANTAGONISTS, BPH, "ZOSINS"
   TERAZOSIN

JNC-8/ACC
1. THIAZIDE
2. ACE/ARB
3. CCB(DHP)
4. β-BLOCKER
5. ALDO-A

COMORBID CONDITIONS

BRADYCARDIA, BLUNT HYPO

$$MAP = CO \times$$
$$HR \times SV$$
$$CONT \times$$

β₁ HEART COMPENSATORY
β₁ + β₂ PROPRANOLOL OR NADOLOL
(NONSELECTIVE) ASTHMA, ED, ψ ↓
ESOPHAGEAL VARICES, HEMORRHAGE PPX

β₁ METOPROLOL (PO, IV) ESMOLOL (IV GTT)
CAD, HFrEF
+RATE CONTROL

β₁-α₁ CARVEDILOL AND LABETALOL
CAD, HFrEF IV +
+ BP CONTROL PO TID ESRD

OD = GLUCAGON

ATI	ACE-I "-PRILS"	ANGIOEDEMA DRY COUGH ↓ Ø	↑Cr↑K		CHF CAD
	ARB "-ARTON"		↑Cr↑K̄ TERATOGENIC		CMD OM ETC. HTN
CC	DHP-CCB "-DIPINES"	PERIPHERAL EDEMA	—		ANTIANGINAL
NO	ARTERIES HYDRALAZINE	REFLEX TACHY	DRUG-INDUCED LUPUS	IV + (HR <90)	

SVR = AFTERLOAD
α-SNS ATI- AngZ ... NO₁ ARTERIAL CALCIUM CHANNELS

VOLUME, Na, ALDOSTERONE ... NO VENOUS

PL

Na⁺ THIAZIDE DIURETICS HCTZ + CHLORTHALIDONE ↓K, PANCREATITIS HELP Ca OXALATE STONES
LOOP DIURETICS FUROSEMIDE + TORSEMIDE ↓K↓Mg OTOTOXICITY ↓VOL
↳ VOL OVERLOAD (CHF, ASCITES)

ALDO ALDOSTERONE ANTAGONISTS SPIRONOLACTONE + EPLERENONE ↑K
↳ VOL OVERLOAD (CHF, ASCITES) ↳ GYNECOMASTIA ↑Cr

NO NITRATES
ISMN HTN, CAD, ANTIANGINAL HEADACHE PDE5-I
ISDN CHF, BIDIL® ↓BP

Shock

IF ↓ CO ...↑SVR
· ↓SYS WHOMP ↓SYS } NARROW
· ↑DIA BP ↑DIA } PP
· EXTREMITIES COLD

IF ↓ SVR ...↑CO
· ↑SYS WHOMP ↓SYS } WIDENED
· ↓DIA BP ↓DIA } PP
· EXTREMITIES WARM

· FRANK HYPOTENSION MAP < 60
· SHOCK INDEX HR/SYS > 1
· RELATIVE ↓BP · LACTIC ACID ↑ ... FAILS TO CLEAR

INOCONSTRICTOR
SEPSIS
SPINAL TRAUMA
ANESTHESIA
ANAPHYLAXIS
ADDISONS VASOCONSTRICTOR

$$MAP = CO \times SVR$$
TOO FAST
TOO SLOW HR × SV
CONT × PL
↓ EF, MI
INODILATOR

VOL ↓
DIURESIS
DIARRHEA
DEHYDRATION
HEMORRHAGE

OBSTRUCTION
PE
TPTX
PT

VOLUME, BLOOD

SYS BP

↑SVR
↓SVR

DIA BP

DISTRIBUTIVE

HYPOVOLEMIC
OBSTRUCTIVE
CARDIOGENIC

α₁
VASOCONSTRICTORS
PHENYLEPHRINE
VASOPRESSIN
EPINEPHRINE

β₁, α₁
INOCONSTRICTOR
NOREPI
DOPAMINE
↓
SEPTIC SHOCK

β₁, β₂
INODILATOR
DOBUTAMINE
MILRINONE
↓
CHF SHOCK

α₁   β₁   β₂

NOTES

Vasculitis

GCA
PATH: LARGE VESSELS
ART: EXT CAROTID
  OPHTH
>50 TEMPORAL
PT: JAW CLAUDICATION
  VISION CHANGES
  TEMPORAL TENDERNESS

DX: BX

TX: STEROIDS

TAKAYASU
PATH: LARGE VESSELS
ART: AORTA
  +
  BRANCHES
<40
PT: PULSELESSNESS

DX: ANGIOGRAM

TX: STEROIDS

PAN
PATH: HEPB
ART: GUT
  RENAL
  SKIN
PT: MESENTERIC
  ISCHEMIA
  RENAL FAILURE
  PURPURA
  MONONEURITIS
  MULTIPLEX
DX: ANGIOGRAM
TX: STEROIDS
  +
  CYCLOPHOSPHAMIDE

WEGNERS
PATH: ANCA
ART: SMALL
  VESSEL

PT: HEMOPTYSIS
  HEMATURIA
  NOSE

DX: C-ANCA
  BX BEST
TX: STEROIDS
  +
  CYCLOPHOSPHAMIDE

CRYO
PATH: HEP C

PT: PURPURA
  PALPABLE
  +
  HEP C

DX: ↓ COMPLIMENT
  CRYOGLOBULINS

TX: SEVERE: PLASMA
  UNDERLYING DZ
  STEROIDS
  +
  CYCLOPHOSPHAMIDE

HSP
PATH: –

PT: PURPURA
  PALPABLE
  +
  GI
  PAIN BLEED

BX

STEROIDS

Anatomy of the Heart

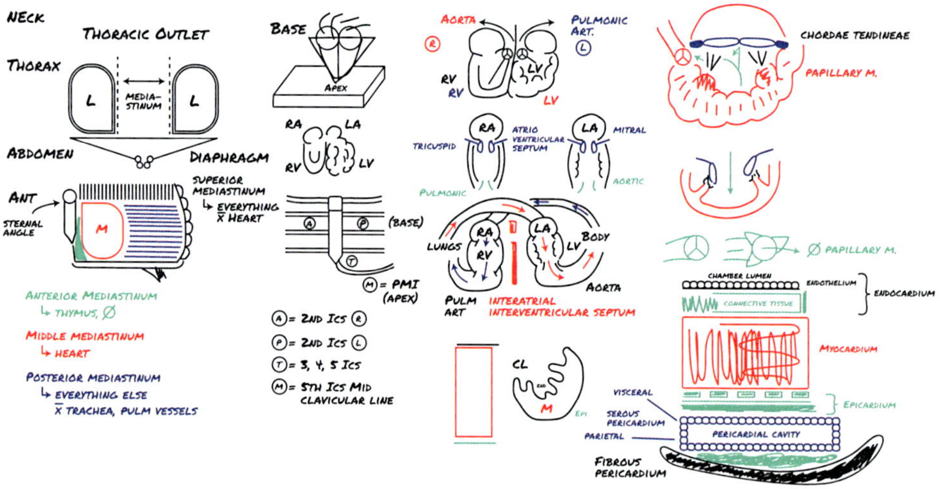

Cardiac

Endocarditis

OnlineMedEd

ENDOCARDIUM

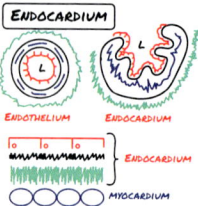

ENDOTHELIUM ENDOCARDIUM

ENDOCARDIUM

MYOCARDIUM

ENDOTHELIUM INJURY + REPAIR

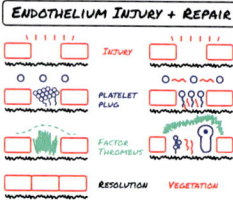

INJURY

PLATELET PLUG

FACTOR THROMBUS

RESOLUTION VEGETATION

INFECTIOUS ENDOCARDITIS

PATH : 90% (L) SIDED ←
- IF (R) SIDED = IVDA, IF IVDA
  EATING VALVES, CHORDAE

DX : "DUKE CRITERIA"
- CULTURE, CULTURE, CULTURE
- TTE → TEE
- PROXIMAL VALVE

TX : IV ABX × 6 WEEKS
- SURGERY IF...
  - FUNGAL   · ≥ 15 CM
  - EMBOLIZATION · FAILED ABX

F/U : "BAD VALVE"
PPX : AMOXICILLIN (STREP)
- BAD VALVE + DIRTY PROCEDURE

NON-INFECTIOUS ENDOCARDITIS

MARANTIC
DEBILITATED, MALNOURISHED +
HYPERCOAGULABLE (CANCER)
NON-DESTRUCTIVE
NON-INFECTIOUS
⊕ THROMBOTIC... EMBOLIZE ⊕ SX
⊕ ANTICOAGULATE
PROXIMAL SIDE VALVES
MULTIPLE + SMALL VEGETATIONS

LSE = SLE
STEROIDS = ↓ INCIDENCE
VEGETATIONS ON BOTH
SIDES OF MITRAL VALVE
NON-DESTRUCTIVE
NON-INFECTIOUS
⊕ ANTICOAGULATE
(APUA)

ACUTE INFECTIOUS BACTERIAL ENDOCARDITIS

PATH : VIRULENT + DESTRUCTIVE BUGS STAPH AUREUS
- AFFECT NORMAL VALVES + REGURGITATION
- OVERT, OBVIOUS ⊕ SX
PT : HIGH-SPIKING FEVERS
- REGURGITANT MURMUR (NEW)
- LARGE VEGETATIONS → SEPTIC EMBOLI
- ⊕ CX... FAILS TO CLEAR

DX : CULTURES EASY, LARGE = TTE
TX : VANCOMYCIN ─── NAFICILLIN
     (MRSA)   (MSSA)

SUBACUTE INFECTIOUS BACTERIAL ENDOCARDITIS

PATH : INSIDIOUS ORGANISMS, NON-DESTRUCTIVE, HACEK
- SUBTLE, INFLAMMATION, "BAD VALVE"
PT : GRADUAL, SUBACUTE, SMOLDERING INFLAMMATION
- ↑ESR, ↑CRP WEIGHT ↑TEMP
              LOSS

MICROEMBOLI

SPLINTER   JANEWAY
HEMORRHAGES   LESIONS
(NAILS)   (PALMS/SOLES)

IMMUNE COMPLEX
VASCULITIS

OSLER   ROTH
NODES   SPOTS
(TIPS DIGITS) (RETINA)

DX : CULTURE A LOT WITHOUT ABX
     ⊖ TTE → ⊕ TEE
TX : CX

Pericardial Disease

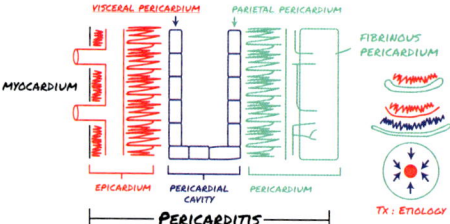

MYOCARDIUM

VISCERAL PERICARDIUM PARIETAL PERICARDIUM

FIBRINOUS PERICARDIUM

EPICARDIUM PERICARDIAL CAVITY PERICARDIUM

TX : ETIOLOGY

── PERICARDITIS ──

ACUTE PERICARDITIS

PATH : MISNOMER — SOME Ø CELLS
- VARIABLE CAUSES, VARIABLE PRESENTATIONS
PT : ① SHARP CP, PLEURITIC, POSITIONAL
     ② TRIPHASIC FRICTION RUB
     ③ DIFFUSE ST-SEGMENT ELEVATIONS

DX : ECG
     -ECHO -MRI

TX : COLCHICINE + NSAIDS
     PREDNISONE

MAIN
CAUSES : VIRAL   POST-INFARCT
          UREMIC   INTRA-INFARCT
          SEROSITIS (SLE)
          CANCERS

SUBTYPES

- SEROUS
- NORMAL FLUID
  VIRAL
- FIBRINOUS
  FIBRINOUS EXUDATE
  POST-INFARCT (4-6 DAYS)
  INTRA-INFARCT (4-6 DAYS)
  CARDIAC SURGERY
- SUPPURATIVE
  INFXN = PUS

          CONSTRICTIVE
          PERICARDITIS
- HEMORRHAGIC

PERICARDIAL EFFUSION

PATH : ↑FLUID IN THE CAVITY
- PERICARDITIS
- PUS (INFXN), FREE WALL RUPTURE
PT : Ø FRICTION RUB
- DYSPNEA PAINLESS
- ↓ HEART SOUNDS
DX : ECG = ELECTRICAL ALTERNANS
- X-RAY = WATER-BOTTLED
- CT/MRI = SEE
- (ECHO) = POCUS
- PERICARDIOCENTESIS

CONSTRICTIVE PERICARDITIS

PATH : REPEATED FIBRINOUS
       OR
       SUPPURATIVE
- RIGID SCARRED PERICARDIUM
PT : "RESTRICTIVE PHYSIOLOGY"
- PERICARDIAL KNOCK
- KUSSMAUL SIGN
- H/O PERICARDITIS
DX : ECG
- X-RAY = CALCIFICATIONS
- ECHO = R/O EFFUSION
- (MRI)
TX : PERICARDIECTOMY

TAMPONADE

PATH : HEMODYNAMIC COMPROMISE
- IMPAIRED RV FILLING DIA
PT : BECK'S TRIAD
     → HYPOTENSION
     → MUFFLED ♡ SOUNDS
     → JVD
DX : PULSUS PARADOXUS > 10 MMHG
- ECHO = ONLY FLUID
TX : EMERGENCY PERICARDIOCENTESIS

EFFUSION TX

① PERICARDIOCENTESIS
NEEDLE, DRAIN FLUID
TAMPONADE, ETIOLOGY

② PERICARDIAL WINDOW
RECURRENT/REFRACTORY
EFFUSIONS
HOLE IN PERICARDIUM

③ PERICARDIECTOMY
REMOVAL OF PERICARDIUM

NOTES

Heart as a Muscle

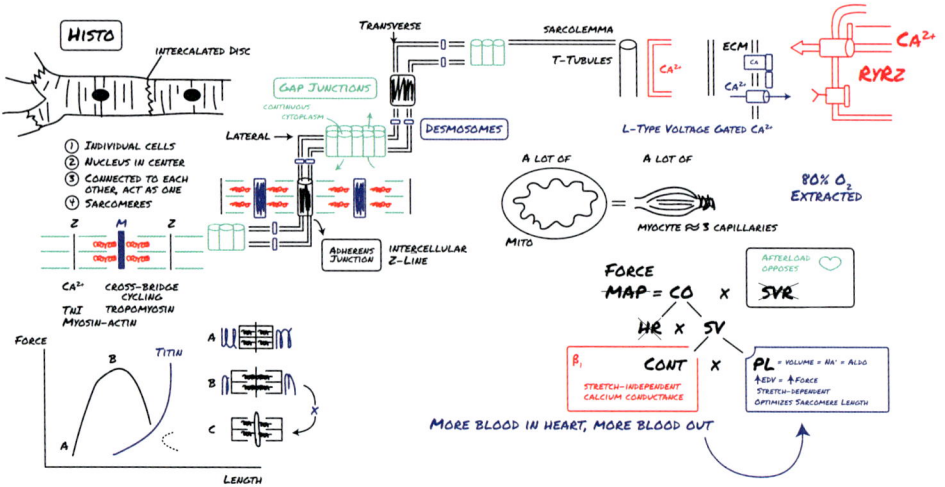

Myocardial Work

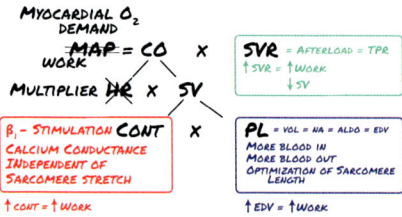

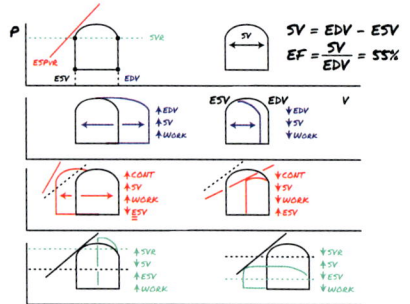

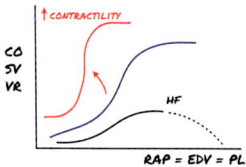

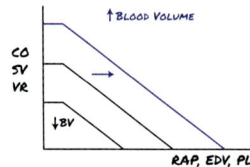

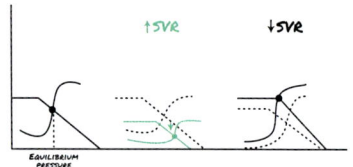

NOTES

Heart Failure

OnlineMedEd

WORK
MAP = CO × SV × CONT

AFTERLOAD = TPR
α₋SNS   ATI = ANGZ
SVR
CONCENTRIC HYPERTROPHY
HFPEF = DIA CHF

VOLUME = NA⁺ = ALDO = EDV
ECCENTRIC HYPERTROPHY
PL
HFREF = SYS CHF

β₁ − STIMULATION
CALCIUM CONDUCTANCE
"COMPENSATORY"
HR

β₁ − STIMULATION = ↑CONT, ↑WORK... TROPHIC SIGNAL (GROW)
↑SVR = ↑AFTERLOAD, ↑WORK.... ALTERS GENE EXPRESSION
↑PL = ↑MAP, ↑WORK... STRETCH... ALTERS GENE EXPRESSION

VENTRICULAR RESPONSE
HYPERTROPHY = HEAVIER
↑AFTERLOAD = CONCENTRIC HYPERTROPHY = STRONGER
IMPAIRED RELAXATION
IMPAIRED FILLING = DIA
EF − , ↑
↑PRELOAD = STRETCH = ECCENTRIC HYPERTROPHY = LONGER
IMPAIRED CONTRACTION
IMPAIRED EMPTYING = SYS
EF↓

JVD   PULMONARY EDEMA = CRACKLES   ANGZ
ANP = BNP   DOE AND ORTHOPNEA
CONGESTIVE HEPATOPATHY
NUTMEG LIVER CIRRHOSIS   DEPENDENT PERIPHERAL EDEMA   WEIGHT GAIN   ALDO
(HOW) BOWEL EDEMA → IV TO TREAT

CELL'S RESPONSE
HYPERTROPHY = ADD SARCOMERE
↑SARCOMERE = ↑WORK
↑WORK ... 5 ↑BLOOD VESSELS
MYOCYTES APOPTOSE
FIBROSIS

SYS vs. DIA
SYS = ↓EF
LEAKY (VALVE INSUFF)
FLOPPY (DILATION)
DEAD (INFARCTION)
S₁ S₂ S₃
DIA = ↓COMPLIANCE
HTN HEART
AORTIC STENOSIS
INFILTRATION
S₄ S₁ S₂

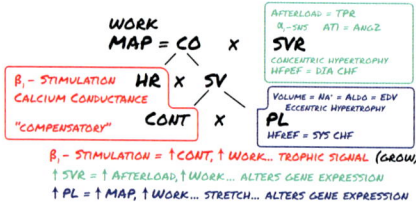

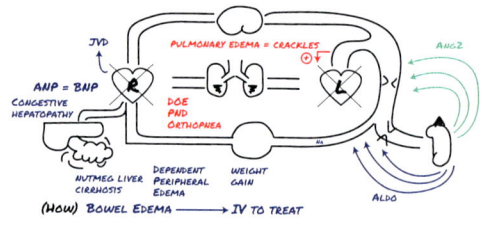

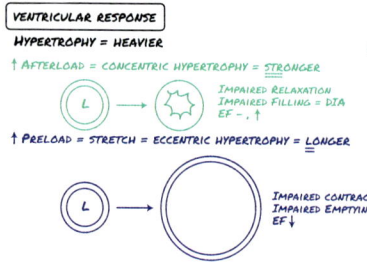

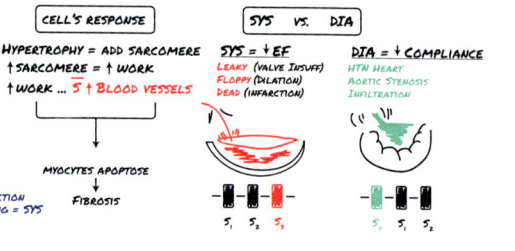

Heart Failure Pharmacology

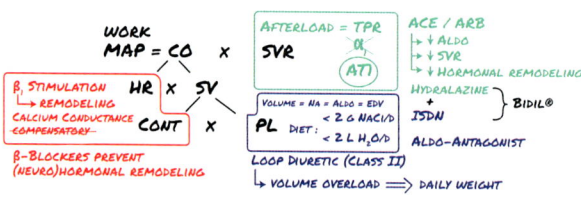

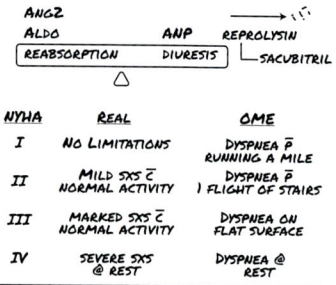

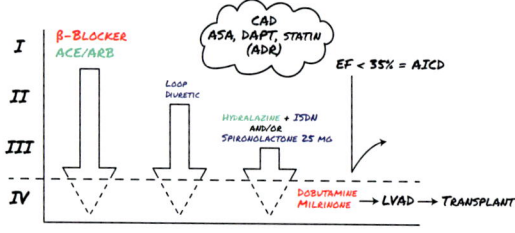

WORK
MAP = CO × SV × CONT
HR

β₁ STIMULATION
↳ REMODELING
CALCIUM CONDUCTANCE
COMPENSATORY
β−BLOCKERS PREVENT
(NEURO)HORMONAL REMODELING

AFTERLOAD = TPR
α
SVR ATI

VOLUME = NA = ALDO = EDV
PL DIET: < 2 G NACl/D
< 2 L H₂O/D
LOOP DIURETIC (CLASS II)
↳ VOLUME OVERLOAD ⟹ DAILY WEIGHT

ACE / ARB
↳ ↓ALDO
↳ ↓SVR
↳ ↓HORMONAL REMODELING
HYDRALAZINE
+
ISDN } BIDIL®
ALDO−ANTAGONIST

ANGZ
ALDO   ANP   REPROLYSIN
REABSORPTION DIURESIS ↳ SACUBITRIL

NYHA	REAL	OME
I	NO LIMITATIONS	DYSPNEA p̄ RUNNING A MILE
II	MILD SXS c̄ NORMAL ACTIVITY	DYSPNEA p̄ ↑ FLIGHT OF STAIRS
III	MARKED SXS c̄ NORMAL ACTIVITY	DYSPNEA ON FLAT SURFACE
IV	SEVERE SXS @ REST	DYSPNEA @ REST

β−BLOCKER ACE/ARB
LOOP DIURETIC
CAD
ASA, DAPT, STATIN (ADR)
HYDRALAZINE + ISDN AND/OR SPIRONOLACTONE 25 MG
EF < 35% = AICD
DOBUTAMINE MILRINONE → LVAD → TRANSPLANT
I II III IV

HFPEF 2/2 HTN
↳ TX HTN
HFPEF 2/2 SOMETHING
↳ ↓HR
AVOID DEHYDRATION

24

© 2021 OnlineMedEd

Cardiac

Cardiomyopathy

DCM

ALL 4 CHAMBERS DILATED
↓ EF
∅CAD

PATH: ALL 4 CHAMBERS DILATED

ECCENTRICITY HYPERTROPHY AND ↓EF

CAUSE: AUTOSOMAL DOM = TITIN DEF.
ALCOHOL ⎱ WET
B₁ DEFICIENCY ⎰ BERI BERI
* COXSACKIE A
CHAGAS
COCAINE
DOXORUBICIN ⎱ DOSE-DEPENDENT
DAUNORUBICIN ⎰ IRREVERSIBLE
TRASTUZUMAB - DOSE INDEPENDENT
IS REVERSIBLE
* PERIPARTUM CARDIOMYOPATHY *

TXI: HFREF ⟶ TRANSPLANT

HOCM

ASYMMETRIC SEPTAL HYPERTROPHY
H/O SUDDEN CARDIAC DEATH
YOUNG SYNCOPE

PATH: ASYMMETRIC SEPTAL ↑ HYPERTROPHY
↓
OUTFLOW OBSTRUCTION

CAUSE: AD MUTATION OF SARCOMERE GENES

PT: VARSITY (YOUNG) ATHLETE SYNCOPAL VOL ↓
• H/O ANKLE SUDDEN CARDIAC DEATH
• "AORTIC STENOSIS"

GROSS: SEPTAL HYPERTROPHY

HISTO: MYOCYTE DISARRAY
SARCOMERE ⟶ ^
FIBROSIS

TX: AVOIDING DEHYDRATION, ↓HR

RESTRICTIVE CM

SPECKLED PATTERN
HIGH PRESSURE, LOW VOL
↑ EF

PATH: INFILTRATION
STIFF VENTRICLE
IMPAIRED FILLING DIA

CAUSES: SARCOID
AMYLOID
HEMOCHROMATOSIS
CANCERS
FIBROSIS (LOEFFLER'S)

PT: ↑ EF USUALLY > 70%
UP TO 90%

GROSS: NO HYPERTROPHY
NO DILATION
INFILTRATION

HISTO: NORMAL MYOCYTES
+ EXTRA STUFF

TAKOTSUBO

OLD FEMALE c̄ CAD RF
p̄ EMOTIONAL STRESS
⊕ STEMI ⟶ CLEAN CORONAVIRUS
APICAL BALLOONING

MYOCARDITIS

VIRAL (COXSACKIE A)
LYMPHOCYTES DCM

↑TROPONINS, ∅ST Δs
YOUNG, ∅RF

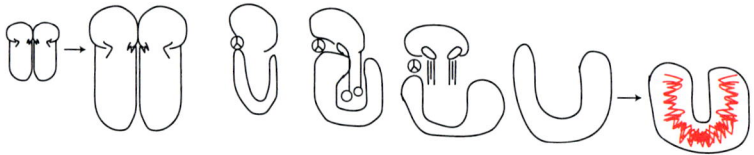

Embryogenesis and Fetal Flow

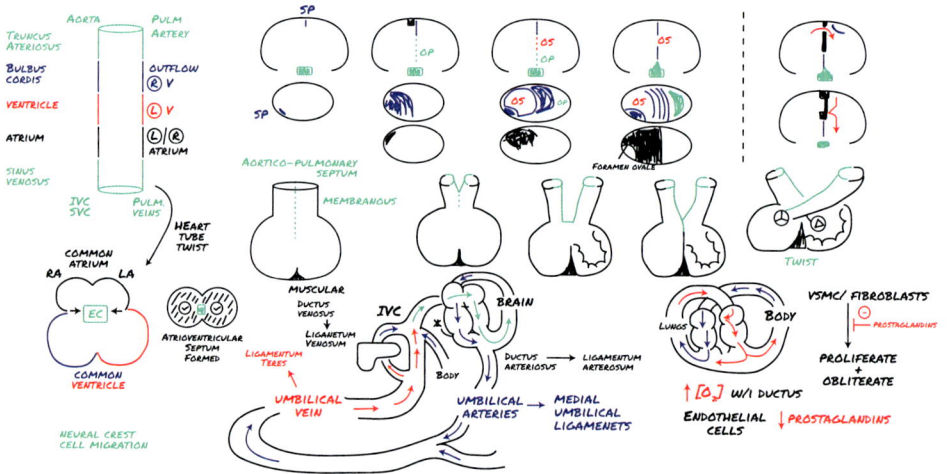

Cardiac

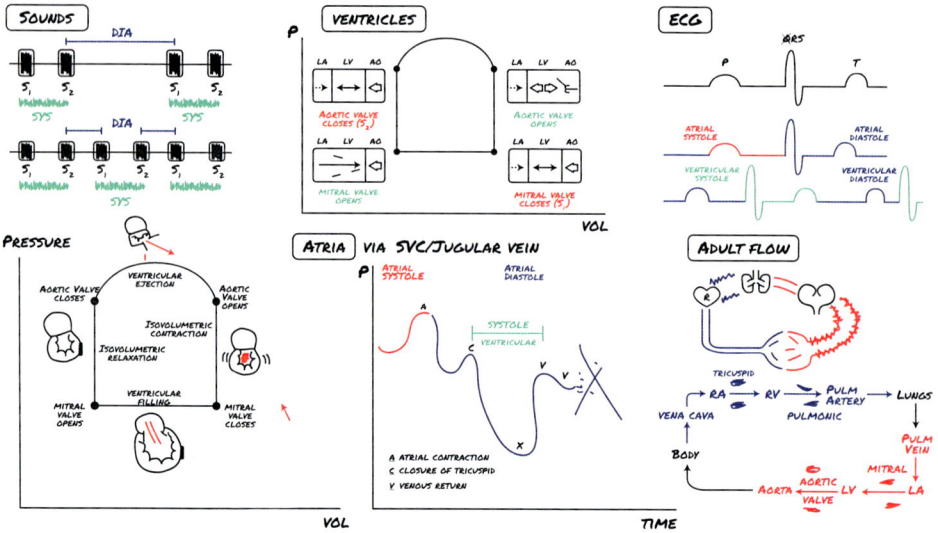

Cardiac Cycle

OnlineMedEd

Valves

VALVE = MURMUR

$$\text{TURBULENCE} = \frac{\text{FLOW}}{\text{AREA}}$$

ATRIA = DILATE

VENTRICLES — CONCENTRIC / ECCENTRIC

AORTIC VALVE — DIA = CLOSING (REGURGITATION) / SYS = OPENING (STENOSIS)

MITRAL VALVE — DIA = OPENING (STENOSIS) / SYS = CLOSING (REGURGITATION)

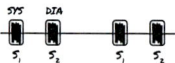

(R) SQUATTING, LEG LIFT ↑PL = ↑MURMUR
VALSALVA = ↓PL = ↓MURMUR

(L) HAND GRIP = ↑SVR

MITRAL STENOSIS
DIA MURMUR, APEX
CAUSE: RHD
ECHO: ↓VALVE AREA
↑PRESSURE GRADIENT

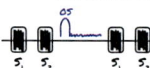

AORTIC STENOSIS
SYS MURMUR
LV CONCENTRIC
CONCENTRIC HYPERTROPHY
CAUSE: RHD
AGE
PT: OLD WHITE MALE
c̄ RF CAD
EXERTIONAL SXS

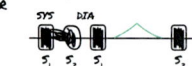

MITRAL INSUFFICIENCY
SYS MURMUR
LA DILATION
CAUSES: ① ENDOCARDITIS
② INFARCTION
③ DCM
↓ LA DILATION

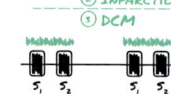

AORTIC INSUFFICIENCY
DIA MURMUR
LV DILATION
↑SYS / ↓DIA — WIDENED PULM PRESSURE

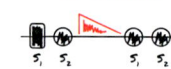

HOCM = "AORTIC STENOSIS"
↑IMPROVES c̄ PC

MVP = MITRAL REGURG
IMPROVES ↑PC

28

© 2021 OnlineMedEd

Cardiac

Noncyanotic Congenital Heart Disease

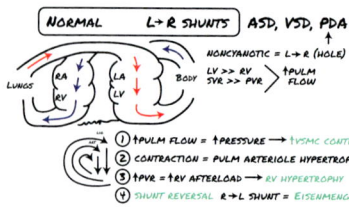

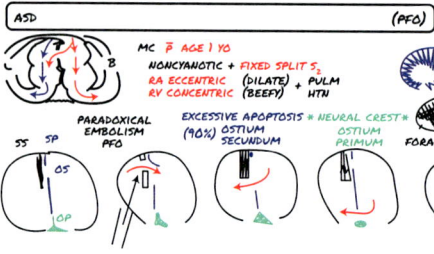

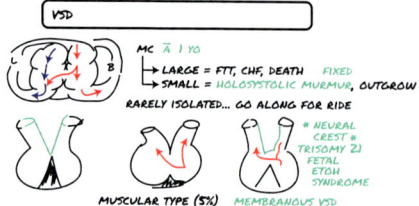

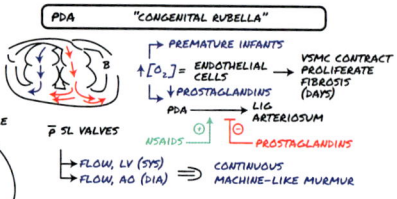

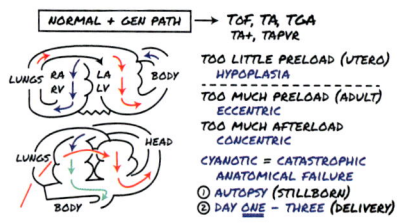

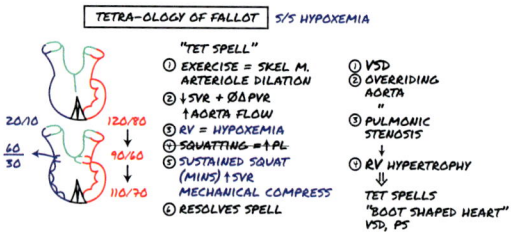

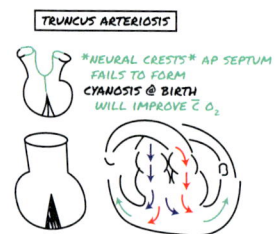

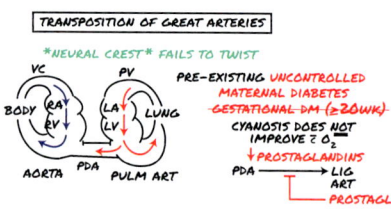

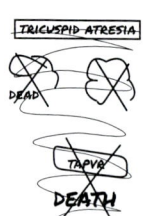

NORMAL | L→R SHUNTS | ASD, VSD, PDA

NONCYANOTIC = L→R (HOLE)

LV >> RV   ↑PULM FLOW
SVR >> PVR

LUNGS RA LA   BODY
RV LV

① ↑PULM FLOW = ↑PRESSURE → ↑VSMC CONTRACTION
② CONTRACTION = PULM ARTERIOLE HYPERTROPHY → ↑PVR
③ ↑PVR = ↑RV AFTERLOAD → RV HYPERTROPHY ⟶ CYANOSIS
④ SHUNT REVERSAL R→L SHUNT = EISENMENGER'S ⟶ CLUBBING ⟶ POLYCYTHEMIA

ASD   (PFO)

MC ≥ AGE 1 YO
NONCYANOTIC + FIXED SPLIT S₂
RA ECCENTRIC (DILATE) + PULM HTN
RV CONCENTRIC (BEEFY)

PARADOXICAL EMBOLISM PFO
EXCESSIVE APOPTOSIS * NEURAL CREST *
(90%) OSTIUM SECUNDUM
OSTIUM PRIMUM
FORAMEN OVALE

SS   SP
OS
OP

VSD

MC ≤ 1 YO
⟶ LARGE = FTT, CHF, DEATH   FIXED
⟶ SMALL = HOLOSYSTOLIC MURMUR, OUTGROW

RARELY ISOLATED... GO ALONG FOR RIDE

* NEURAL CREST *
TRISOMY 21
FETAL ETOH SYNDROME

MUSCULAR TYPE (5%)   MEMBRANOUS VSD

PDA   "CONGENITAL RUBELLA"

⟶ PREMATURE INFANTS
↑[O₂] = ENDOTHELIAL CELLS ⟶ VSMC CONTRACT, PROLIFERATE, FIBROSIS (DAYS)
↓PROSTAGLANDINS "
PDA ⟶ LIG ARTERIOSUM

≥ SL VALVES
NSAIDS ⊣ ⟶ PROSTAGLANDINS

⟶ FLOW, LV (SYS) ⟹ CONTINUOUS
⟶ FLOW, AO (DIA)   MACHINE-LIKE MURMUR

Cyanotic Congenital Heart Disease

NORMAL + GEN PATH → TOF, TA, TGA
TA+, TAPVR

LUNGS RA LA BODY
RV LV

LUNGS   HEAD

BODY

TOO LITTLE PRELOAD (UTERO)
HYPOPLASIA

TOO MUCH PRELOAD (ADULT)
ECCENTRIC
TOO MUCH AFTERLOAD
CONCENTRIC

CYANOTIC = CATASTROPHIC ANATOMICAL FAILURE
① AUTOPSY (STILLBORN)
② DAY ONE – THREE (DELIVERY)

TETRA-OLOGY OF FALLOT S/S HYPOXEMIA

"TET SPELL"
① EXERCISE = SKEL M. ARTERIOLE DILATION
② ↓SVR + ØPVR ↑AORTA FLOW
③ RV = HYPOXEMIA
④ SQUATTING = ↑PL
⑤ SUSTAINED SQUAT (MINS) ↑SVR MECHANICAL COMPRESS
⑥ RESOLVES SPELL

20/10   120/80
60/30   90/60
          110/70

① VSD
② OVERRIDING AORTA
   "
③ PULMONIC STENOSIS
④ RV HYPERTROPHY

TET SPELLS
"BOOT SHAPED HEART"
VSD, PS

TRUNCUS ARTERIOSIS

NEURAL CRESTS AP SEPTUM FAILS TO FORM
CYANOSIS @ BIRTH
WILL IMPROVE ē O₂

TRANSPOSITION OF GREAT ARTERIES

NEURAL CREST FAILS TO TWIST

VC   PV
BODY RA PV LUNG
RV LV

AORTA PDA PULM ART

PRE-EXISTING UNCONTROLLED MATERNAL DIABETES
~~GESTATIONAL DM (≥20WK)~~
CYANOSIS DOES NOT IMPROVE ē O₂
↓PROSTAGLANDINS
PDA ⊣ LIG ART
⟶ PROSTAGLANDIN

TRICUSPID ATRESIA

DEAD

TAPVR

DEATH

Cardiac

Coronary Vessels and Cardiac Conduction

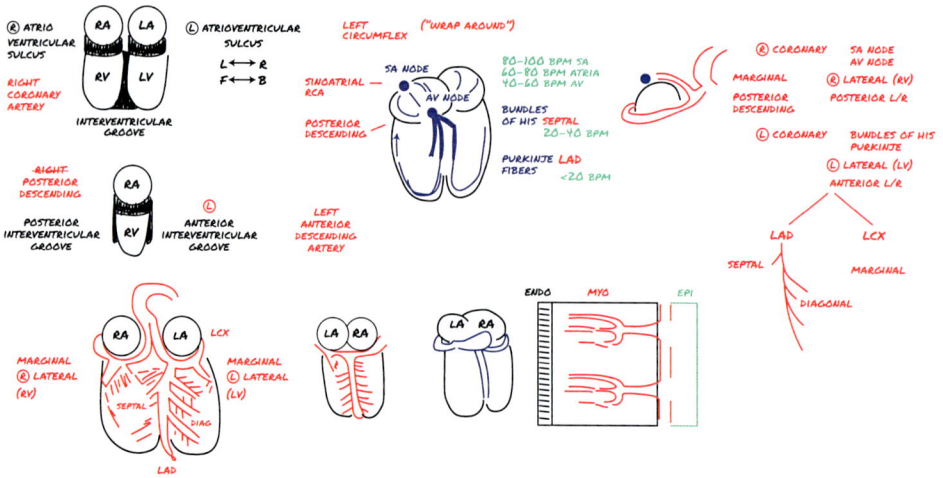

® ATRIO VENTRICULAR SULCUS

RIGHT CORONARY ARTERY

INTERVENTRICULAR GROOVE

Ⓛ ATRIOVENTRICULAR SULCUS

L ⟷ R
F ⟷ B

SINOATRIAL — RCA

POSTERIOR DESCENDING

RIGHT POSTERIOR DESCENDING

POSTERIOR INTERVENTRICULAR GROOVE

Ⓛ ANTERIOR INTERVENTRICULAR GROOVE

LEFT CIRCUMFLEX ("WRAP AROUND")

SA NODE

AV NODE

80-100 BPM SA
60-80 BPM ATRIA
40-60 BPM AV

BUNDLES OF HIS SEPTAL 20-40 BPM

PURKINJE FIBERS LAD <20 BPM

LEFT ANTERIOR DESCENDING ARTERY

® CORONARY   SA NODE / AV NODE
MARGINAL   ® LATERAL (RV)
POSTERIOR   POSTERIOR L/R
DESCENDING
Ⓛ CORONARY   BUNDLES OF HIS PURKINJE
              Ⓛ LATERAL (LV)
              ANTERIOR L/R

LAD   LCX
SEPTAL   MARGINAL
  DIAGONAL

MARGINAL ® LATERAL (RV)

SEPTAL   DIAG

LAD

LCX

MARGINAL Ⓛ LATERAL (LV)

ENDO   MYO   EPI

Conduction System

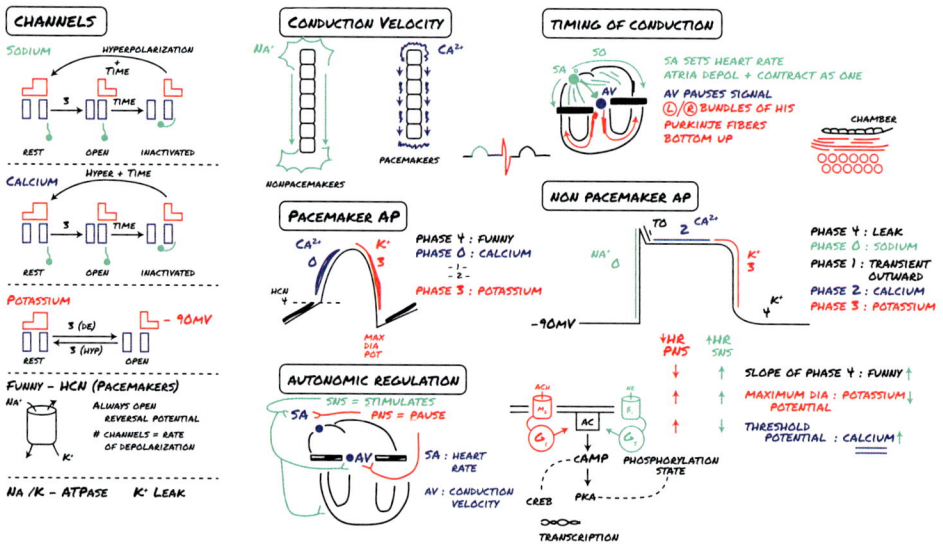

CHANNELS

SODIUM

REST   OPEN   INACTIVATED

CALCIUM

REST   OPEN   INACTIVATED

POTASSIUM   −90MV

REST   OPEN

FUNNY − HCN (PACEMAKERS)
ALWAYS OPEN
REVERSAL POTENTIAL
CHANNELS = RATE OF DEPOLARIZATION

NA /K − ATPASE   K⁺ LEAK

CONDUCTION VELOCITY

NA⁺   CA²⁺

NONPACEMAKERS   PACEMAKERS

PACEMAKER AP

CA²⁺   K⁺

HCN

MAX DIA POT

PHASE 4 : FUNNY
PHASE 0 : CALCIUM
PHASE 3 : POTASSIUM

AUTONOMIC REGULATION

SNS = STIMULATES
PNS = PAUSE

SA : HEART RATE

AV : CONDUCTION VELOCITY

TIMING OF CONDUCTION

SA SETS HEART RATE
ATRIA DEPOL + CONTRACT AS ONE
AV PAUSES SIGNAL
Ⓛ/® BUNDLES OF HIS
PURKINJE FIBERS
BOTTOM UP

CHAMBER

NON PACEMAKER AP

T0   2 CA²⁺

NA⁺ 0   K⁺ 3

−90MV   K⁺ 4

PHASE 4 : LEAK
PHASE 0 : SODIUM
PHASE 1 : TRANSIENT OUTWARD
PHASE 2 : CALCIUM
PHASE 3 : POTASSIUM

↑HR PNS   ↑HR SNS

SLOPE OF PHASE 4 : FUNNY
MAXIMUM DIA : POTASSIUM POTENTIAL
THRESHOLD POTENTIAL : CALCIUM

ACH   AC   β

cAMP   PHOSPHORYLATION STATE

CREB   PKA

TRANSCRIPTION

Cardiac

Visualizing the EKG

OnlineMedEd

RHYTHM STRIP

P-WAVE | R QRS COMPLEX | T-WAVE
PR SEGMENT | ST SEGMENT
PR INTERVAL
QT INTERVAL

ATRIAL DEPOL | REPOL BURIED QRS | REPOL
VENTRICULAR DEPOL

ATRIAL SYSTOLE | ATRIAL DIA

VENT DIA | VENT SYS

SA NODE | AV NODE | BUNDLES
"ATRIAL KICK" | PURKINJE FIBERS

AMPLITUDE — FORCE / MASS + DIRECTION / MEMBRANE POTENTIAL

EKG INTERPRETATION
1. REGULAR OR IRREGULAR?
2. RATE = # QRS x TIME 300 150 100 75 60 50
3. QRS WIDE OR NARROW? ≥ 120   < 120
4. P FOR EVERY QRS
5. QRS FOR EVERY P
6. PR INTERVAL < 200

USING T-WAVES
NORMAL
ISCHEMIA "FLIPPED T"
ST SEGMENT ELEVATION INFARCTING
INFARCTING
INFARCTED Q WAVE
OLD INFARCT

12 LEAD "SEPTAL" = SEPTUM SEPTAL
I –
II –
III AVF
"INFERIOR" = RV POSTERIOR DESCENDING

V1 | V4
V2 | V5
V3 | V6

"ANTERIOR" = LV LEFT ANTERIOR DESCENDING
"LATERAL" = LV LEFT CIRCUMFLEX

AXIS DEVIATION = ROCKETSHIP
E L R
I:↓ AVF:↓ EXTREME AXIS DEVIATION
I:↑ AVF:↓ AXIS DEVIATION
I:↓ AVF:↑ AXIS DEVIATION (UP)
I:↑ AVF:↑ NORMAL (DOWN)

USING P-WAVES
NORMAL (SA) | JUNCTIONAL (AV) | ATRIAL | VENTRICLES

HYPERTROPHY
1. BEST = ECHO / POCUS
2. INAPPROPRIATE TOUCHING V1-V4 BUT NOT ELSEWHERE
3. BOXES

[V1 OR V2] + [V5 OR V6] ≥ 35
V1 | V4
V2 | V5
V3 | V6

Arrhythmias

SINUS BRADYCARDIA < 60
NORMAL SINUS RHYTHM
SINUS TACHYCARDIA > 100
NOT ARRYTHMIAS

SLOW BLOCK ← ARRHYTHMIA → FAST REENTRY / FIBRILLATION

BRADY IS HEART BLOCK
"BLOCK" = IMPAIRED CONDUCTION AV NODE INFARCTION OR INFILTRATION

1° FIXED PROLONGED PR INTERVAL (≥200)
2° TYPE I: PROLONGING OF PR INTERVAL c̄ DROPPED QRS
2° FIXED II: PR FIXED RANDOM DROPS
3° AV DISSOCIATION (A) (V)

SUPRAVENTRICULAR TACHYCARDIA
AVNRT | AVRT=WPW | A. FLUTTER | A. FIB >300
CONDUCTION VELOCITY
MONOMORPHIC V. TACH

VENTRICULAR TACHYCARDIAS
MONOMORPHIC V. TACH | POLYMORPHIC = TORSADES V. TACH ECTOPI
V. FIB
ASYSTOLE = DEAD

34

© 2021 OnlineMedEd

Cardiac

Anti-Arrhythmics

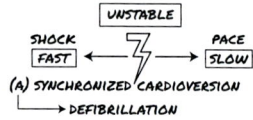

CLASS I
SODIUM CHANNELS
NON-PACEMAKERS

IA REST OPEN (K)
IB INACTIVATED
IC ACC

NEVER USE

QUINIDINE
PROCAINAMIDE (PROLONG QT)

LIDOCAINE = SEIZURE
MEXILETINE

FLECAINIDE
PROPAFENONE

CLASS II BETA-BLOCKERS
PACEMAKERS = RATE CONTROL
NONPACEMAKERS = ↓CONTRACTILITY
↑ECTOPI
↓MI

↑K ↓HCN ↓CA

→ HFrEF + EXACERBATION
AFIB ≳ RUN = CONTRAINDICATION

CLASS III
POTASSIUM BLOCKERS
NON-PACEMAKERS

AMIODARONE
SOTALOL

CLASS IV
CALCIUM BLOCKERS

↓AUTOMATICITY
↓CONDUCTION VELOCITY

→RATE CONTROL←
NON - DHP
VERAPAMIL
DILTIAZEM

PACEMAKERS

NON-PACEMAKERS ↓CONTRACTILITY

UNCLASSIFIED

ADENOSINE — BREAK REENTRY CIRCUIT OR SLOW TO SEE

DIGOXIN — AFIB ≳ RVR + HFrEF EXACERBATION
GOOD GFR

MG — TORSADES

BRADYCARDIA

M₂-ANTAG
ATROPINE-
PREPARE TO PACE

ACH
AC
cAMP
PKA
↓K ↑FUNNY ↑CA

β₁-AGONISTS
EPINEPHRINE
DOPAMINE
DOBUTAMINE

UNSTABLE

SHOCK
FAST

PACE
SLOW

(A) SYNCHRONIZED CARDIOVERSION
→ DEFIBRILLATION

Pathophysiology of Atherosclerosis

"SCLEROSIS"
- ARTERI-O-SCLEROSIS
  ↳ VAGUE, "NARROWING" "HARDENING"
- MONCKEBERG MEDIAL SCLEROSIS
  ↳ CALCIFICATION OF TUNICA MEDIA
  ↳ NO NARROWING OF LUMEN
- HYPERPLASTIC ARTERIOL-O-SCLEROSIS
  ↳ MALIGNANT HTN
  ↳ CONCENTRIC MEDIA ≳ REDUPLICATION OF THE ELASTIC LAMINA
- HYALINE ARTERIOL-O-SCLEROSIS
  ↳ HTN, DM → LEAKY ENDOTHELIUM
  ↳ THICKENED BM

ATHEROSCLEROSIS
↳ OCCURS IN LARGE ELASTIC AND MEDIUM MUSCULAE ARTERIES
↳ ATHEROMA = PLAQUE
↳ ECCENTRIC COMPROMISE OF LUMEN EVENTUALLY CHRONIC ISCHEMIA
↳ RUPTURES = THROMBOSIS ACUTE ISCHEMIA

CVD (TIA) → CVA
CAD (SA) → MI
PVD (CLAUDICATION) → ALI

ANATOMY OF PLAQUE
MEDIA
MYOFIBROBLASTS
FIBROUS CAP
MYOFIBROBLASTS (COLLAGEN)
NECROTIC LIPID CORE (LDL, CHOLESTEROL, FOAM)

RISK FACTORS
MODIFIABLE — NONMODIFIABLE
DM   OBESITY   M > 45 FAM HX
HTN SMOKING   F > 55 GENETICS
HLD   *AGE*

INITIATION OF PLAQUE
① ENDOTHELIAL DYSFXN = LEAKY
   ↳ FATTY STREAKS FOUND IN TEENAGERS @ BRANCHPOINTS
   ↳ TURBULENT FLOW (HEMODYNAMIC STRESS)
② LDL DEPOSITS
   ↳ LDL TO EXIT ENTER INTIMA
   ↳ LDL IS OXIDIZED
   ↳ IMMUNE SYSTEM RESPONDS
   ENDOTHELIUM LEAKY
   MACROPHAGES ENGULF LDL
   CYTOKINES + LDL
   FOAM CELLS NECROSIS

PROGRESS
FATTY STREAK
BIGGER LUMEN / THIN MEDIA — ARTERIAL REMODELING
LUMEN COMPROMISED — COMPLEX ATHEROMA
MYOFIBROBLAST COLLAGEN — FIBRO FATTY PLAQUE
SXS ≳ EXERTION — STABLE PLAQUE + CRITICAL STENOSIS (>70%)
BRUIT — COLLATERALS
UNSTABLE PLAQUE — RUPTURE IS THROMBOSIS

HEMODYNAMIC STRESS
ENDOTHELIAL DYSFXN
LIPID CORE { LDL ENTERS INTIMA / LDL OXIDIZES

ENDOTHELIAL CELLS "HELP!"
MACROPHAGES → FOAM CELLS → DIE
NECROTIC LIPID CORE { NECROTIC FOAM CELLS / LDL OXIDIZES
PDGF = TUNICA MEDIA PROLIFERATION

MYOFIBROBLASTS PROLIFERATE IN MEDIA → TUNICA INTIMA TO LAY COLLAGEN
SHIELD THROMBOGENIC CORE FROM CIRCULATING FACTORS
FAILS TO PREVENT CYCLE
↑LDL ↑FOAM NECROSIS
↑PDGF ↑MYOFIBROBLAST

↑TURBULENT FLOW
↑LDL ↑FOAM
↑PDGF ↑MYOFIBROBLAST

RATIO CORE: CAP WORSE OVERTIME
MMPS PERMITS REMODELING
MMPS 2/2 MACROPHAGES NECROSIS
MATRIX DEGENERATION ←

Cardiac

Pharmacology of Atherosclerosis

③ CIRCULATING LDL

BILE ACID RESIN, EZETIMIBE
⊣
ABSORPTION

LDL-R   oPCSK9 ⊣ PCSK9-I

↓DIETARY
CHOLESTEROL
+
FAT

① DIET

● LDL
=●= IDC
BODY

HMG-COA
REDUCTASE
VLDL
STATINS

② DE NOVO
SYNTHESIS

FIBRATES
GEMFIBROZIL FENOFIBRATE
LIGANDS FOR PPARα
* ↓TRIGLYCERIDES *
FAMILIAL
HYPERTRYGLYCERIDEMIA

LIPOPROTEIN
LIPASE
ENDOTHELIAL

HEPATOTOXIC
MYOPATHY

PPARα

ADIPOCYTE

* STATINS * + DIET

HIGH-POTENCY ROSUVASTATIN 20, 40
              ATORVASTATIN 40, 80
HMG-COA-REDUCTASE-I = ⇧LDL-R
SE: HEPATOTOXICITY + MYOPATHY

PCSK9 - INHIBITORS

MONOCLONAL AB vs PCSK9 = ⇧LDL-R
EVOLOCUMAB, ALIROCUMAB
INJECTABLE : INFLAMMATION @ SITE
    -MAB : FLU-LIKE REACTION
IND : MAX STATIN + NEW VASCULAR
      STATIN INTOLERANCE

BILE ACID RESINS

BIND TO AND INHIBIT BILE ACIDS
PREVENT:
① BILE ACID REABSORPTION (MADE IN LIVER)
② LIPID DIGESTION
③ LIPID ABSORPTION
④ CHOLESTEROL ABSORPTION
⑤ CHOLESTEROL REABSORPTION ┘ (WASTE)
RESULTS: ⇧⇧LDL-R
COLESTIPOL CHOLESTYRAMINE

STEATORRHEA
ADEK DEFICIENCIES
MED MALABSORPTION

EZETIMIBE

BINDS TO CHOLESTEROL
① —
② —   DIARRHEA
③ —   NOT
              AS BAD   → NON-ADHERENCE
④ CHOLESTEROL ABSORPTION
⑤ CHOLESTEROL REABSORPTION
RESULT: ↑ LDL-R

NIACIN
↑HDL
FLUSHING
PPX ASA

GLUCOSE
DHAP

HORMONE
SENSITIVE
LIPASE

c c c

TRIGLYCERIDES

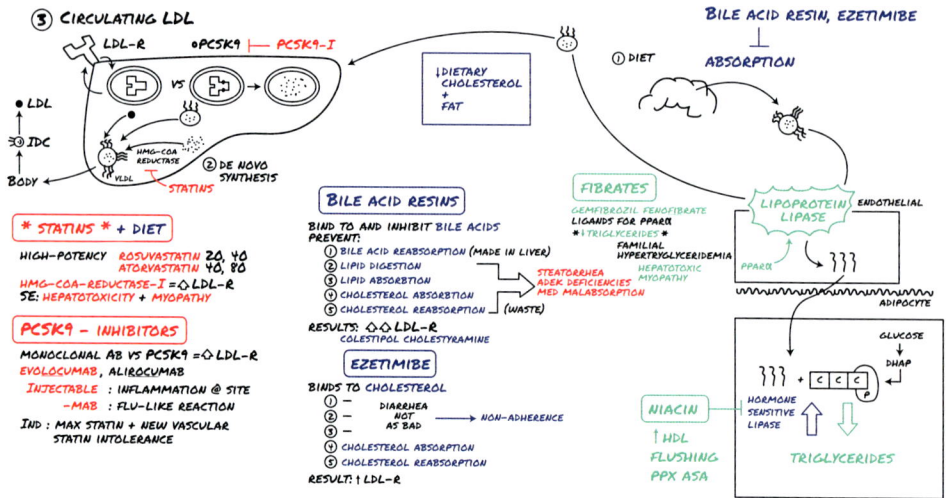

Chronic Ischemic Heart Disease

DEMAND VS. SUPPLY

DEMAND = STABLE PLAQUE
·△ IN MYOCARDIAL O₂ DEMAND
    ↑ AFTERLOAD (SVR)
    ↑ HR
    ↑ CONTRACTILITY
    "↑ PRELOAD" - NTG ↓PL
·∅ACUTE △ IN VESSEL DIAMETER
    - CRITICAL STENOSIS ⊙
    - NOT A △... NOT ACUTE

SUPPLY = RUPTURED + THROMBOSIS

⊙△VESSEL DIAMETER
100% = STEMI
≤ 100% = UA, NSTEMI

- - - - - - - - - - - - - - - -
↓DO₂ = "SUPPLY"
GLOBAL HYPOTENSION
↓ [O₂]
OTHER

IS IT ANGINA?

INTRAPERSON = FIXED
INTERPEOPLE = VARIABLE
① DIAMOND - FORRESTER
   -SUBSTERNAL CRUSHING
   =
   * WORSENS ₹ EXERTION
   * IMPROVES ₹ NTG
② ASSOCIATED SXS
   PRESYNCOPE NAUSEA
   DYSPNEA   DIAPHORESIS
③ RISK FACTORS
   DM OBESITY M > 45
   HTN SMOKING F > 55
   HLD   FAM HX
                AGE
④ PHYSICAL
   NONTENDER
   NONPOSITIONAL
   NONPLEURITIC
⑤ LABS
   TROPONIN-1 ⎫
   12-LEAD   ⎬ SETTING
   A1C (DM)   ⎭
   TSH
   LIPID

MAKING THE DIAGNOSIS

STRESS   TEST
TREADMILL   ECG
PHARMA   ECHO
              NUCLEAR

GOAL: ⇧ DEMAND
   PROVOKES 5X
   VISUALIZES DZ

12-LEAD: ST △S
ECHO:

REST
NORMAL   RISK   SCAR
⊕   ∅   ∅
STRESS

⊖ STRESS ≠ ⊖ CAD
⊖ STRESS = ⊖ ≥70%
⊕ STRESS → CATH

ONLY
ANGIOGRAM = LHC
R/I OR R/O

FIX ONLY > 70%

CORONARY STEAL

DIPYRIDAMOLE = SUPPLY

PRINZMETAL'S ANGINA

SUPPLY ISCHEMIA 2/2

ACUTE ↓LUMINAL DIAMETER
NOT THROMBOSIS

VASOSPASM... DRUGS
· TRIPTANS
· COCAINE   ⎱ ⇧MYOCARDIAL
· AMPHETAMINE ⎰   O₂ DEMAND
YOUNG, ₹ R/F, ⊕STEMI
CLEAN CORONARIES

NOTES

Chronic Ischemic Heart Disease Pharmacology

ALL CAD : ASA STATIN ACE-I BETA-BLOCKER + DAPT

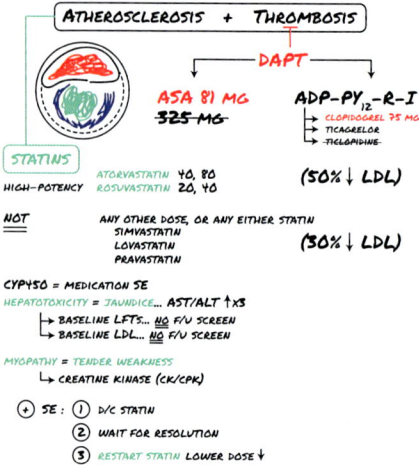

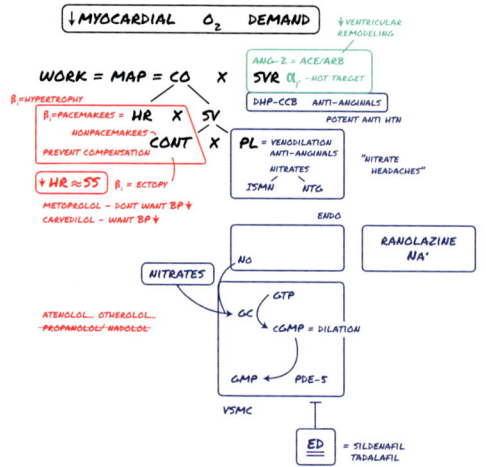

ATHEROSCLEROSIS + THROMBOSIS

DAPT

ASA 81 MG
~~325 MG~~

ADP-PY$_{12}$-R-I
→ CLOPIDOGREL 75 MG
→ TICAGRELOR
→ ~~TICLOPIDINE~~

(50% ↓ LDL)

STATINS

HIGH-POTENCY   ATORVASTATIN 40, 80
                ROSUVASTATIN 20, 40

<u>NOT</u>   ANY OTHER DOSE, OR ANY EITHER STATIN
           SIMVASTATIN
           LOVASTATIN   (30% ↓ LDL)
           PRAVASTATIN

CYP450 = MEDICATION SE

HEPATOTOXICITY = JAUNDICE... AST/ALT ↑X3
  → BASELINE LFTS... <u>NO</u> F/U SCREEN
  → BASELINE LDL... <u>NO</u> F/U SCREEN

MYOPATHY = TENDER WEAKNESS
  → CREATINE KINASE (CK/CPK)

(+) SE : ① D/C STATIN
         ② WAIT FOR RESOLUTION
         ③ RESTART STATIN LOWER DOSE ↓

↓ MYOCARDIAL O$_2$ DEMAND   ↓ VENTRICULAR REMODELING

WORK = MAP = CO   X   SVR   ANG-2 = ACE/ARB
                              α$_1$ - NOT TARGET

β$_H$=HYPERTROPHY   DHP-CCB   ANTI-ANGINALS
  β$_1$=PACEMAKERS → HR X SV   POTENT ANTI HTN
  NONPACEMAKERS →
PREVENT COMPENSATION   CONT X   PL = VENODILATION
                                      ANTI-ANGINALS   "NITRATE
↓ HR ≈ 55   β$_1$ = ECTOPY   NITRATES   HEADACHES"
                                    ISMN   NTG
METOPROLOL - DON'T WANT BP ↓
CARVEDILOL - WANT BP ↓

                                              ENDO
                              NITRATES   RANOLAZINE
                                        NO   NA⁺
ATENOLOL... OTHEROLOL...   GTP
~~PROPANOLOL~~ ~~NADOLOL~~   GC
                                    cGMP = DILATION

                              GMP   PDE-5

                              VSMC

                              ED   = SILDENAFIL
                                      TADALAFIL

Acute Coronary Syndrome

ACUTE CORONARY SYNDROMES

THROMBOSIS = SUPPLY ISCHEMIA

	UA WORSENING	NSTEMI REST	STEMI REST
PAIN			↗
TROPS	⊖	⊕	... ↗
ST ↑	⊖	⊖	
% OCC	>70%	>90%	100%
INFARCT	⊖	⊕	⊕

TRANSMURAL VS. SUBENDOCARDIAL

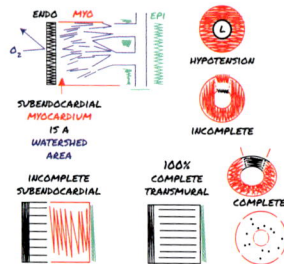

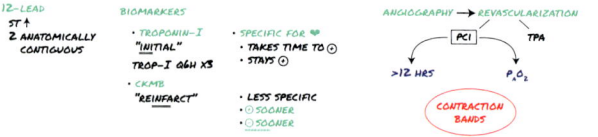

ENDO MYO   EPI

O$_2$

HYPOTENSION

SUBENDOCARDIAL
MYOCARDIUM
IS A
WATERSHED
AREA

INCOMPLETE

100%
COMPLETE
TRANSMURAL

INCOMPLETE
SUBENDOCARDIAL

COMPLETE

TIME	PHASE	HISTOLOGY	GROSS	COMPLICATIONS
< 4 HRS	EARLY REVERSIBLE LATE REVERSIBLE NECROSIS	NORMAL	NORMAL	CARDIOGENIC SHOCK ARRHYTHMIA
4 HRS - 24 HRS	COAGULATIVE NECROSIS	WAVY MYOCYTES ↓ INTENSE EOSINOPHILIA	RED	ARRHYTHMIA
1 D - 3 D	EARLY INFLAMMATORY PHASE	NEUTROPHILS + MYOCYTES	YELLOW PALLOR	FIBRINOUS PERICARDITIS
4 D - 7 D	LATE INFLAMMATORY PHASE	MACROPHAGES	YELLOW PALLOR	RUPTURE (3 D - 7 D) – FREE WALL – SEPTUM – PAPILLARY M.
7 D - 14 D	PROLIFERATIVE PHASE	FIBROBLASTS ANGIOGENESIS LOOSE COLLAGEN CT	PALLOR SOFTENS	
14 D - 28 D	MATURATION PHASE	FIBROBLAST DENSE COLLAGEN CT	GREY	DRESSLER SYNDROME (AI PERICARDITIS)
28+ D	COMPLETION	↓ ACELLULAR SCAR	BRIGHT WHITE	ANNEURYSM → MURAL THROMBUS

12-LEAD
ST ↑
2 ANATOMICALLY
CONTIGUOUS

BIOMARKERS
• TROPONIN-I
  "INITIAL"
  TROP-I Q6H X3
• CKMB
  "REINFARCT"

• SPECIFIC FOR ❤
• TAKES TIME TO ⊕
• STAYS ⊕

• LESS SPECIFIC
  ⊕ SOONER
  ⊖ SOONER

ANGIOGRAPHY → REVASCULARIZATION

                    PCI   TPA
              >12 HRS   P$_{x}$O$_2$

              CONTRACTION
              BANDS

Cardiac

Pharmacology of ACS

OnlineMedEd

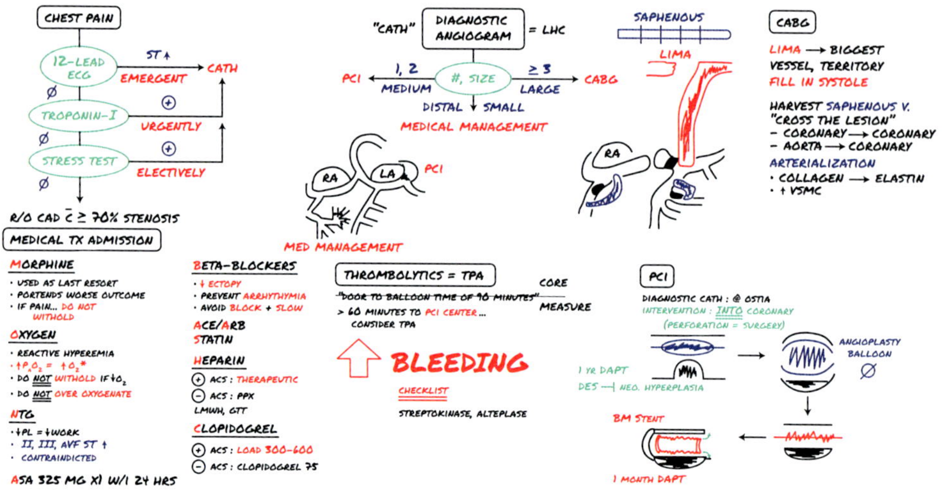

Cardiac

OnlineMedEd

ROTATOR CUFF

↑ SUPRASPINATUS — ABDUCT 0°-15° SUPRASCAPULAR N.
↓ INFRASPINATUS — EXTERNAL SUPRASCAPULAR N.
POSTERIOR TERES MINOR — ROTATION AXILLARY

- - - -

ANTERIOR SUBSCAPULARIS — INTERNAL ROTATION SUBSCAPULAR N.

FOREARM = EXTRINSIC MUSCLES OF HAND
ANTERIOR "FLEXORS" ULNAR N. MEDIAN N.
POSTERIOR "EXTENSORS" RADIAL N.

HAND

5 4 3 2

HYPOTHENAR
PINKY
"DIGITI MINIMI"
ULNAR N.

THENAR
THUMB
"POLLICIS"
MEDIAN N.

LUMBRICALS
FLEX MCP
EXTEND DIP, PIP
4,5 = ULNAR N.
1,2 = MEDIAN N.
INTEROSSEI DAB-PAD
DORSAL ABDUCT
PALMAR ADDUCT
ULNAR N.

DIP
PIP
MCP

T T C
S L T P

SCAPHOID
LUNATE
TRIQ
PIRIFORM
HAMATE
CAPITATE
TRAPS
TRAPS

NOT ROTATOR CUFF

DELTOID — ABDUCTION 15°-100° AXILLARY
TRAPEZIUS — ABDUCTS > 90° CNXI
SERRATUS ANT — ABDUCTS > 100° LONG THORACIC
LATS — EXTEND SHOULDER THORACODORSAL, INT ROTATE, ADDUCT —
PECS — FLEX SHOULDER

ARM
BICEPS — FLEX ELBOW, PRONATE FOREARM
TRICEPS — EXTEND ELBOW, SUPINATE

AXILLARY
BRACHIAL
RADIAL
ULNAR

ACROMION
CLAVICLE
CORACOID
HUMERUS
SCAPULA
LATERAL
MEDIAL CONDYLE
EPICONDYLE
ANNULAR LIGAMENT
RADIUS
ULNA
CARPAL
METACARPAL
PHALANGES

ROTATOR CUFF

DEFECT = WEAKNESS
PT C/O = PAIN...

S UPRA SPIN — AB 0°-15° EMPTY CAN DROP ARM
I NFRA SPIN — EXTERNAL ROTATION LAG TEST
T x

- - - -

S UBSCAP — INTERNAL ROTATION LAG TEST

TENDINITIS
TENDINOPATHY
TENDON RUPTURE

LOSE N. INNERVATES = NO PAIN MUSCLE LESION

IMPINGEMENT = PAIN

SHOULDER DISLOCATIONS

ELBOW ADDUCTED
ANTERIOR
EXTERNALLY ROT
ANY TRAUMA, COMMON
AXILLARY N. → DELTOID ATROPHY PARESTHESIAS

POSTERIOR
INTERNALLY ROT
LIGHTNING, SEIZURES

ELBOW

LATERAL EPICONDYLITIS
ORIGIN: EXTENSORS
PAIN/TENDER LAT
RESIST FLEXION
TENNIS ELBOW

MEDIAL EPICONDYLITIS
ORIGIN: FLEXORS
PAIN/TENDER MED
RESIST EXTENSION
GOLFER'S ELBOW

RADIAL HEAD SUBLUXATION
ANNULAR LIGAMENT
KIDS GET YANKED
FLEXED, INT ROTATED
PAIN @ ELBOW

WRIST

CARPAL TUNNEL
MEDIAN N.
COMPRESSION

THENAR PAIN
ATROPHY PARESTHESIA
SPARING THENAR (LATE)
EMINENCE TINEL, PHALEN
RF → NSAIDS → SPLINT → CUT

HAND, FRACTURES

BOXER'S FX = BARE KNUCKLE FIGHTER, HIT A WALL

C
T

GREENSTICK

TORUS

AXIAL STRESS

FOOSH

① SCAPHOID FX ADULT
DAY 0: NO DEFORMITY NO X-RAY
DAY 7: PAIN AT SNUFF BOX NECROTIC X-RAY

② RADIAL HEAD FX
ELDERLY ♀
OSTEOPOROSIS
WRIST PAIN
COLLES (EXT)
SMITH (FLEX)

③ SUPRACONDYLAR HUMERUS
MC FX KIDS
GROWTH PLATE
PAIN @ ELBOW

ULNAR N. COMPRESSION

CYCLIST
HYPOTHENAR ATROPHY
PAIN
PARASTHESIA
WEARING GLOVES

NOTES

Nerves of the Upper Extremity

MOTOR

| ANTERIOR FOREARM | FLEXORS | MEDIAN ULNAR |
| POSTERIOR FOREARM | EXTENSOR | RADIAL |

THENAR	THUMB	MEDIAN
HYPOTHENAR	PINKY	ULNAR
INTEROSSEI	DAB-PAD	ULNAR
LUMBRICALS	FLEX MCP	1,2,3-M
	EXT DIP/PIP	4,5-U

HUMERAL FX

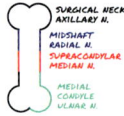

- SURGICAL NECK / AXILLARY N.
- MIDSHAFT / RADIAL N. / SUPRACONDYLAR MEDIAN N.
- MEDIAL CONDYLE / ULNAR N.

CUTANEOUS - TERMINAL

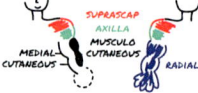

- SUPRASCAP
- AXILLA
- MUSCULO CUTANEOUS
- MEDIAL CUTANEOUS
- RADIAL

MOTOR - TERMINAL

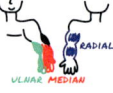

- RADIAL
- ULNAR MEDIAN

CUTANEOUS - DERMATOME

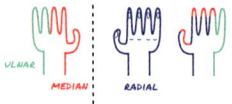

ULNAR   MEDIAN   RADIAL

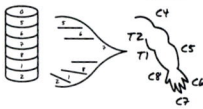

C4, T2, T1, C8, C7, C5, C6

TERMINAL N. LESIONS

PROXIMAL RADIAL	CRUTCHES BARSTOOLS	WRIST DROP / POSTERIOR SENSATION LOST
PROXIMAL MEDIAN	Fx	"POPE'S BLESSING" / 1,2,3 CANNOT FLEX / REMAIN EXTENDED / WHILE MAKING FIST
DISTAL MEDIAN	Fx	CUTANEOUS PALMAR / LATERAL LOST / 1,2,3 MCP EXT / DIP/PIP FLEXED / @ REST
CARPAL TUNNEL	PAIN PARASTHESIA	
PROXIMAL ULNAR	Fx SURGICAL TABLE	4,5 CANNOT FLEX / REMAIN EXTENDED / WHILE MAKING FIST
DISTAL ULNAR	Fx ULNA	CUTANEOUS PALMAR / MEDIAL LOST / 4,5 MCP EXT / DIP/PIP FLEX / @ REST

INTRA PLEXUS LESIONS

ERB'S PALSY = WAITER'S TIP
UPPER TRUNK C5-C6
CHILDBIRTH, HEAD DISPLACED

SHOULDER	AB	ADDUCTED
	EXT ROT	INT ROT
ELBOW	FLEXION	EXTENDED
FOREARM	SUPINATION	PRONATION

KLUMPKE'S CLAW
LOWER TRUNK C8-T2
CHILDBIRTH, FALLING + CATCHING

LUMBRICAL 1-5 MCP EXT / DIP/PIP FLEXED

+EDEMA/PANCOAST TUMOR → THORACIC OUTLET SYNDROME
CERVICAL

WINGED SCAPULA   SERRATUS
LONG THORACIC N.   ABDUCTION > 100°
LN DISSECTION
AXILLARY

PLEXUS

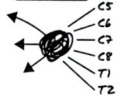

C5, C6, C7, C8, T1, T2

Anatomy of the Lower Extremity

BONES

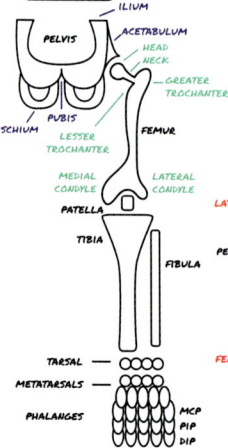

- ILIUM
- PELVIS
- ACETABULUM
- HEAD / NECK
- GREATER TROCHANTER
- PUBIS
- ISCHIUM / LESSER TROCHANTER / FEMUR
- MEDIAL CONDYLE / LATERAL CONDYLE
- PATELLA
- TIBIA
- FIBULA
- TARSAL
- METATARSALS
- PHALANGES / MCP PIP DIP

PERONEAL = LATERAL = FIBULAR

THIGH/PELVIS

GLUTEAL	GLUTEUS MAXIMUS	EXTEND HIP	INFERIOR GLUTEAL N.
LATERAL	GLUTEUS OTHERUS	ABDUCTOR	SUPERIOR GLUTEAL N.
POSTERIOR	"HAMSTRINGS"	FLEX KNEE / EXTEND HIP	SCIATIC N.
MEDIAL	"OBTURATOR"	ADDUCTION	OBTURATOR N.
ANTERIOR	"QUADS"	EXTENDS KNEE / FLEX HIP	FEMORAL N.

FORELEG

ANTERIOR	EXTRINSIC EXTENSORS	DORSIFLEXION / EXTEND TOES / *INVERSION	DEEP PERONEAL N.	ANTERIOR TIBIAL A.
POSTERIOR	EXTRINSIC FLEXORS	PLANTAR FLEXION / FLEX TOES / *INVERSION	*TIBIAL N.	POSTERIOR TIBIAL A.
LATERAL	–	EVERSION	SUPERFICIAL PERONEAL N.	PERONEAL A.

FEMORAL A.
SUPERFICIAL
TIBIAL
DEEP PERONEAL
ANTERIOR TIBIAL
POSTERIOR TIBIAL

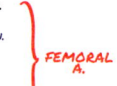

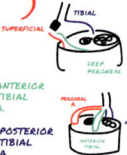

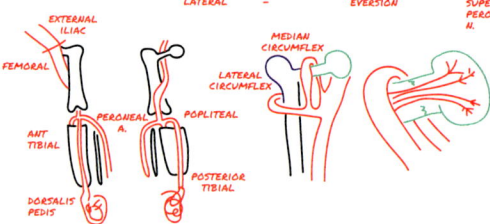

- EXTERNAL ILIAC
- FEMORAL
- MEDIAN CIRCUMFLEX
- LATERAL CIRCUMFLEX
- POPLITEAL
- PERONEAL A.
- ANT TIBIAL
- POSTERIOR TIBIAL
- DORSALIS PEDIS
- WATERSHED AREA / AVASCULAR NECROSIS

Musculoskeletal

Joints of the Lower Extremity

OnlineMedEd

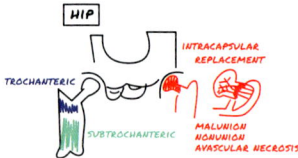

HIP

INTRACAPSULAR REPLACEMENT
TROCHANTERIC
SUBTROCHANTERIC
MALUNION NONUNION AVASCULAR NECROSIS

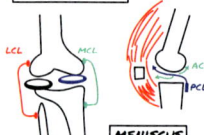

FX	DISLOCATED
SHORTENED	SHORTENED
EXTERNALLY ROTATED	INTERNALLY ROTATED
FEMORAL A.	SCIATIC
FEMORAL N.	

AVASCULAR NECROSIS

CORTICOSTEROIDS, LUPUS
SICKLE CELL DISEASE
GROIN PAIN INABILITY
TO BEAR WEIGHT,
PAIN ₹ USE
X-RAY: CRESCENT (EARLY)
COMPLETE COLLAPSE
FEMUR HEAD Δ5

ANTERIOR TIBIOFIBULAR LIG
HIGH ANKLE SPRAIN
PLANTARFLEXION

ANTERIOR TALOFIBULAR
LOW ANKLE SPRAIN
INVERTED FOOT

TALUS

NORMAL KNEE

LCL MCL
ACL
PCL

MENISCUS

FOOT PLANTED, KNEE ROTATED
(PIVOT)
LOCKING PAIN ₹ PIVOTING
SLOW EFFUSION, CAN WALK
APLEY, MEMORY

TRAUMATIC KNEE

TRAUMA, INABILITY TO WALK
RAPID EFFUSION
MCL VALGUS (VALATERAL) STRESS
SPORT INJURY, TACKLE
MEDIAL LAXITY
LCL VARUS STRESS
CATASTROPHIC
LATERAL LAXITY
PCL DASHBOARD, MVC
POSTERIOR DRAWER
ACL TACKLING, PIVOTING AT HIGH SPEED
ANTERIOR DRAWER (90°)
LACHMAN (30°)

OVERUSE KNEE

① PREPATELLAR BURSITIS
  –HOUSEMAID'S KNEE
  –REPETITIVE KNEELING
  –PAIN @ PATELLA
② PATELLOFEMORAL
  –OVERUSE, RUNNERS
  –PAIN @ TIBIAL TUBEROSITY
  –ADULT BUMP
③ OSGOOD-SCHLATTER'S
  –ADOLESCENTS, ₹ BUMP
  –SQUATS, JUMPING
  –PAIN @ TIBIAL TUBEROSITY
④ ILIOTIBIAL BAND
  –OVERUSE, RUNNERS
  –PAIN @ LATERAL CONDYLE
⑤ BAKER'S CYST
  –POPLITEAL FOSSA
  –U/S ⊖ DVT

SHIN SPLINTS

X-RAY = NORMAL
DEMINERALIZATION
OUTPACES
REMINERALIZATION
CORTEX
VAGUE

STRESS FX

X-RAY = FX, TRAUMA
"FEMALE ATHLETE TRIAD"
  ↳ LOW CALORIE
  ↳ AMENORRHEA
  ↳ LOW BONE DENSITY
VIT D DEFICIENCY
PINPOINT

Nerves of the Lower Extremity

THIGH/PELVIS

GLUTEAL	EXTEND HIP	INF. GLUTEAL
LATERAL	A**B**DUCT	SUP. GLUTEAL
POSTERIOR	HIP EXTENSION KNEE FLEXION	SCIATIC
MEDIAL	ADDUCTS	OBTURATOR
ANTERIOR	HIP FLEXION KNEE EXTENSION	FEMORAL

FORELEG

ANTERIOR	DORSIFLEXION INVERSION
POSTERIOR	PLANTARFLEXION INVERSION
LATERAL	EVERSION

CUTANEOUS-TERMINAL

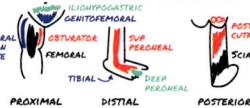

ILIOHYPOGASTRIC
GENITOFEMORAL
OBTURATOR
FEMORAL
LATERAL CUTAN NERVE
SUP PERONEAL
DEEP PERONEAL
TIBIAL
POSTERIOR CUTANEOUS
SCIATIC
PROXIMAL DISTIAL POSTERIOR

CUTANEOUS-DERMATOME

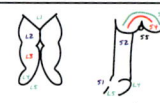

DEEP PERONEAL
TIBIAL
SUP PERONEAL

SECTIONS OF NERVES

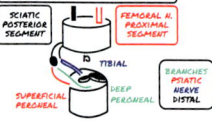

SCIATIC POSTERIOR SEGMENT
FEMORAL N. PROXIMAL SEGMENT
TIBIAL
BRANCHES PSIATIC NERVE DISTAL
SUPERFICIAL PERONEAL
DEEP PERONEAL

HERNIATED DISC (BELOW) →
SPONDYLOSIS

RADICULOPATHY

OSTEOPHYTES →
SPINAL STENOSIS

	L5 LATERAL ANTERIOR	S1 POSTERIOR FORELEG	L2-L4 OBTURATOR FEMORAL
MOTOR LOST	DORSIFLEXION TOE EXTENSION EVERSION	PLANTARFLEXION TOE FLEXION ANKLE JERK	ADDUCT HIP FLEXION KNEE EXTENSION KNEE REFLEX
SENSATION LOST	LATERAL SHIN DORSUM FOOT	BOTTOM OF FOOT	MEDIAL THIGH ANTERIOR THIGH
CANNOT DO	HEEL WALK	TOE WALK	—

NERVE BY NERVE

NERVE	MOTOR	SENSORY	MECHANISM
ILIOHYPOGASTRIC	–	SUPRAPUBIC	TRANSVERSE ABD CLOSED
GENITOFEMORAL	CREMASTER REFLEX	GENITAL SKIN MEDIAL THIGH	OPEN SURGERY RETRACTOR
OBTURATOR	MEDIAL THIGH	MEDIAL THIGH	TROCHAR LAP SURGERY
LATERAL CUTANEOUS	–	LATERAL THIGH	TOO TIGHT CLOTHES OBESE
FEMORAL	ANTERIOR THIGH	ANTERIOR THIGH	PELVIC/HIP FX
SUPERFICIAL PERONEAL	LATERAL FORELEG	ANTERIOR SHIN	FIB FX COMPARTMENT SYNDROME
DEEP PERONEAL	ANTERIOR FORELEG	WEB TOES	"
TIBIAL	POSTERIOR FORELEG	SOLE HEEL	TIB FX
SCIATIC	POSTERIOR THIGH	POSTERIOR FORELEG	POSTERIOR DISLOCATION
POSTERIOR CUTANEOUS	–	POSTERIOR THIGH	–
SUPERIOR GLUTEAL	LATERAL LOCOMOTION	–	POOR IM INJECTION TRENDELENBURG
INFERIOR GLUTEAL	GLUTEAL	–	POSTERIOR DISLOCATION
PUDENDAL	URETHRA + ANUS VALVE	PERINEUM	CHILD BIRTH

48

© 2021 OnlineMedEd

Musculoskeletal

Monoarticular Arthropathy

	APPEARANCE	NORMAL CLEAR	OA CLEAR	INFLAM CLOUDY	SEPTIC OPAQUE
MONOARTICULAR EFFUSION HIGH ACUITY HIGH TOXICITY → ARTHROCENTESIS	WBC	< 200	200-2000	2000-50,000	> 50,000
	OBJECTS	—	—	CRYSTALS	ORGANISMS

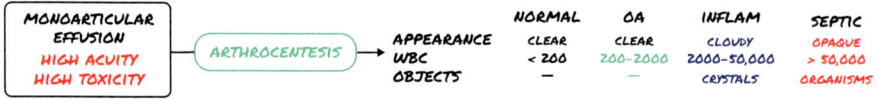

CRYSTAL DEPOSITION GOUT

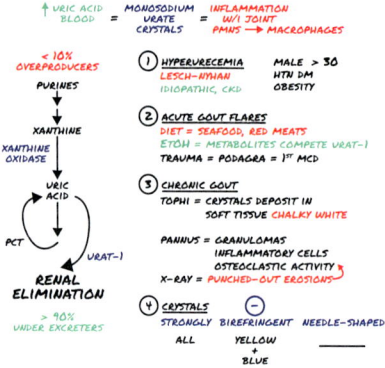

↑ URIC ACID = MONOSODIUM = INFLAMMATION
BLOOD   URATE   W/I JOINT
         CRYSTALS   PMNS → MACROPHAGES

< 10%
OVERPRODUCERS
PURINES

① HYPERURECEMIA   MALE > 30
   LESCH-NYHAN   HTN DM
   IDIOPATHIC, CKD   OBESITY

② ACUTE GOUT FLARES
   DIET = SEAFOOD, RED MEATS
   ETOH = METABOLITES COMPETE URAT-1
   TRAUMA = PODAGRA = 1ST MCD

XANTHINE

XANTHINE
OXIDASE

③ CHRONIC GOUT
   TOPHI = CRYSTALS DEPOSIT IN
           SOFT TISSUE CHALKY WHITE

URIC
ACID

PANNUS = GRANULOMAS
         INFLAMMATORY CELLS
         OSTEOCLASTIC ACTIVITY
X-RAY = PUNCHED-OUT EROSIONS

PCT

URAT-1

RENAL
ELIMINATION
> 90%
UNDER EXCRETERS

④ CRYSTALS ⊖
   STRONGLY BIREFRINGENT NEEDLE-SHAPED
   ALL   YELLOW
              +
              BLUE

PSEUDOGOUT = CPPD

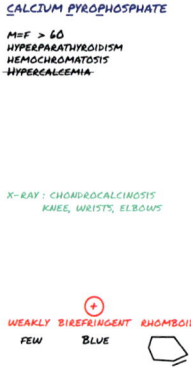

CALCIUM PYROPHOSPHATE

M=F > 60
HYPERPARATHYROIDISM
HEMOCHROMATOSIS
HYPERCALCEMIA

X-RAY : CHONDROCALCINOSIS
        KNEE, WRISTS, ELBOWS

⊕ WEAKLY BIREFRINGENT RHOMBOID
  FEW   BLUE

SEPTIC ARTHRITIS STAPH. AUREUS

PATH: HEMATOGENOUS SPREAD, SKIN TO BLOOD
      ENDOCARDITIS, IVDA, PICC
      PENETRATING INJURIES: PPX WASHOUT
PT: SEPTIC EFFUSION
TAP: > 50,000 WBC   GRAM ⊕ COCCI
      ⊕ ORGANISMS   CLUSTERS
TX: VANCOMYCIN, NAFCILLIN

SEPTIC ARTHRITIS - N. GONORRHEA

PATH: HEMATOGENOUS SPREAD, STI DISSEMINATED
PT: HIGH-RISK SEXUAL BEHAVIOR
      SEPTIC, EFFUSION
TAP: > 50,000 WBC   NAAT
      Ø ORGANISMS → THAYER MARTIN
                    GO LOOKING
TX: CEFTRIAXONE + DOXYCYCLINE

REACTIVE ARTHRITIS

Gout Pharmacology

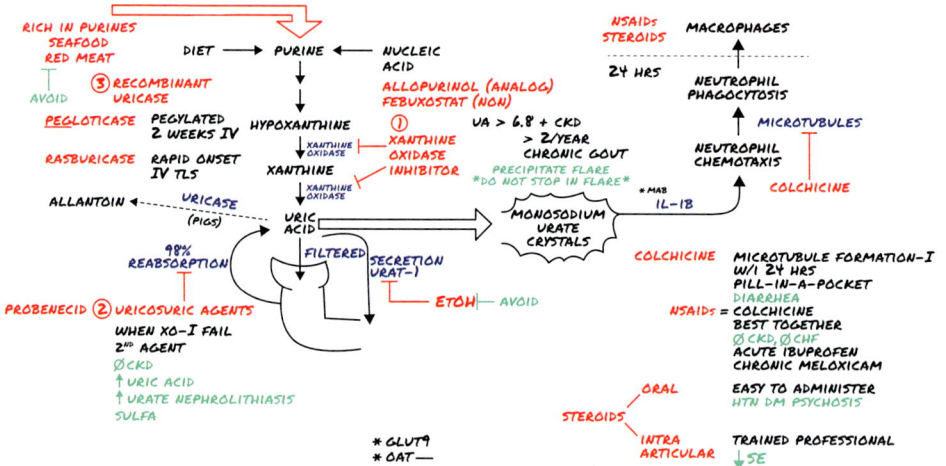

RICH IN PURINES
SEAFOOD
RED MEAT → DIET → PURINE ← NUCLEIC
                            ACID
AVOID ③ RECOMBINANT
         URICASE   ALLOPURINOL (ANALOG)
PEGLOTICASE PEGYLATED   FEBUXOSTAT (NON)
             2 WEEKS IV
                          HYPOXANTHINE   ①
RASBURICASE RAPID ONSET   XANTHINE
             IV TLS   XANTHINE   OXIDASE
                          OXIDASE   INHIBITOR
                          XANTHINE
ALLANTOIN ◄ --- URICASE   XANTHINE
                (PIGS)   OXIDASE
                          URIC
         98%   ACID
      REABSORPTION FILTERED
                          SECRETION
PROBENECID ② URICOSURIC AGENTS URAT-1
             WHEN XO-I FAIL
             2ND AGENT   ETOH ─ AVOID
             Ø CKD
             ↑ URIC ACID
             ↑ URATE NEPHROLITHIASIS
             SULFA

* GLUT9
* OAT ─

NSAIDs
STEROIDS MACROPHAGES

24 HRS   NEUTROPHIL
          PHAGOCYTOSIS

UA > 6.8 + CKD   MICROTUBULES
    > 2/YEAR
CHRONIC GOUT NEUTROPHIL
PRECIPITATE FLARE CHEMOTAXIS
DO NOT STOP IN FLARE   COLCHICINE

MONOSODIUM   * MAB
URATE   IL-1B
CRYSTALS

COLCHICINE MICROTUBULE FORMATION-I
            W/I 24 HRS
            PILL-IN-A-POCKET
            DIARRHEA
NSAIDs   = COLCHICINE
            BEST TOGETHER
            Ø CKD, Ø CHF
            ACUTE IBUPROFEN
            CHRONIC MELOXICAM

ORAL   EASY TO ADMINISTER
STEROIDS HTN DM PSYCHOSIS

INTRA   TRAINED PROFESSIONAL
ARTICULAR ↓ SE

Musculoskeletal

Polyarticular Arthropathies

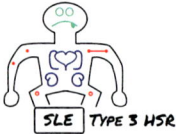

SLE | **TYPE 3 HSR**

PATH: AB–AG COMPLEXES DEPOSIT
+
EARLY COMPLEMENT DEFICIENCY

PT: AA/HISPANIC ♀ REPRODUCTIVE

MALAR RASH
DISCOID RASH

BLOOD – ↓COUNT
RENAL FAILURE
RPGN-2

SEROSITIS ⎯ LSE
⎣ PLEURITIS
⎣ PERICARDITIS

ANA ⊕

ORAL ULCERS
ARTHRITIS, LARGE
PHOTOSENSITIVITY

IMMUNE ⎯ DSDNA
⎣ SMITH
⎣ HISTONE (DRUG)

NEUROLOGIC = ENCEPHALITIS

DX: CLX, INFXN (↑C₄) FLARE (↓C₄)
TX: HYDROXYCHLOROQUINE (1ᵗ)
   MTX, MM, 6-MP (2ᵈ)
   STEROIDS (FLARE)
   CYCLOPHOSPHAMIDE (LUPUS NEPHRITIS)

MORBID: CKD → ESRD
MORTALITY CAD → MI

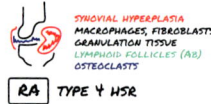

SYNOVIAL HYPERPLASIA
MACROPHAGES, FIBROBLASTS
GRANULATION TISSUE
LYMPHOID FOLLICLES (AB)
OSTEOCLASTS

RA | **TYPE 4 HSR**

PATH: T CELL–MEDIATED PANNUS
+
ANTIBODIES (DX) HLA-DR4

PT: ELDERLY WHITE ♀♂
   FINGER STIFFNESS/DEFORMITY
   > 1 HR MORNING STIFFNESS
   SYMMETRIC MCP PIP

ARTICULAR

SPARES DIP
DEFORMITIES ⎯ SWAN NECK
⎣ ULNAR DEVIATION

EXTRA
ARTICULAR

RHEUMATOID NODULES = FIBRINOID NECROSIS
CARPAL TUNNEL
CERVICAL SUBLUXATION

DX=RF: IgM vs. Fc IgG
CCP= SPECIFIC
XRAY: MARGINAL EROSIONS
   PERIARTICULAR OSTEOPENIA
DX: PANNUS

TX: MTX (1ᵗ LINE)
   TNF-α-I INFLIXIMAB
   ETANERCEPT
   STEROIDS (FLARES)
   NSAIDS (SX CONTROL)

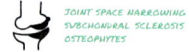

JOINT SPACE NARROWING
SUBCHONDRAL SCLEROSIS
OSTEOPHYTES

OA | **NOT AUTOIMMUNE**

PATH: DAMAGED/LOSS OF CARTILAGE

PT: IMPACT, REPETITIVE USE, OBESITY
   JOINT SURGERY
   PAIN RELIEVED BY REST
   MORNING STIFFNESS < 1 HR

DX: XRAY = ASYMMETRIC
TX: SX → REPLACEMENT

BOUCHARD PIP
HEBER DENS DIP

HAND OA

ASYMMETRIC, DIPS, NO EROSIONS

SERONEGATIVE SPONDYLO | **HLA-B27**

PSORIASIS   PSORIASIS + ARTHRITIS (HANDS)
           Ø AXIAL SKELETON
           NAIL PITTING

ANK   MALES LOW BACK PAIN
SPOND   XRAY = BAMBOO SPINE

IBD-   CROHN'S OR UC + ARTHRITIS
RELATED   TX IBD = TX ARTHRITIS

REACTIVE CAN'T SEE   PEE   CLIMB A TREE
          CONJUNCTIVITIS URETHRITIS ASYMMETRIC
                                      OLIGO
                                      ARTHROPATHY

Other Rheumatologic Conditions

SARCOIDOSIS ?

PATH: ① MACROPHAGE ENGULFS AG
   ② TH0 → TH1
   ③ IFN-γ ACTIVATES MACROPHAGE
   ④ DON'T DIE

NONCASEATING GRANULOMA
ACE ⎣→ 1α-HYDROXYLASE

PT: PULMONARY SARCOID
   A A♀ 20-40 HYPOXEMIA
   B HILAR LYMPHADENOPATHY
   DPLD (ILD)
   EXTRAPULMONARY SARCOID
   HEART = HEART BLOCK, BRADY
   SKIN = LUPUS PERNIO

DX: ACE +,25 VIT·D ↑CA
   X-RAY → BIOPSY

TX: STEROIDS (FLARE)
   O₂

SCLERODERMA

PATH: NON-INFLAMMATORY FIBROBLASTS
   FIBROSIS OF VESSELS
   FIBROSIS OF ORGANS
⎣→ LcSSc = CREST
   SKIN = WRISTS/ANKLES
   CALCINOSIS
   RAYNAUD'S
   G**E**RD
   SCLERODACTYLY
   TELANGIECTASIAS
   ANTI – CENTROMERE
   PULM HTN ∓ HYPOXEMIA
⎣→ DcSSc = "CREST +"
   SKIN = ELBOWS/KNEES
       FACE
   PULM FIBROSIS = ↓O₂
   ANTI-TOPOISOMERASE (SCL 70)
   ANTI-RNA POLYMERASE 3
   SCLERODERMA RENAL CRISIS
   MAHA   STEROIDS
   ↓PLT
   ↑CR   ACE-I
   HTN

SJOGRENS = SICCA SYNDROME

PATH: LYMPHOCYTIC INFILTRATION EXOCRINE
   SALIVARY, TEAR

PT: ♀40-60
ARTIFICIAL → DRY MOUTH → CAVITIES
         → DRY EYES → MALTOMA
   ⓅPAINFUL = PAROTIDITIS   SSA RO
   ⓋPAINLESS = CANCER

DX: ANTI-RIBONUCLEAR PROTEIN-SSB LA
   LOOK FOR ANOTHER DZ

APLA

PATH: ANTI-PHOSPHOLIPID ABS
   IN LAB – ANTICOAGULANT
   IN PERSON – PROCOAGULANT
   LUPUS. 1°, ANOTHER DZ

PT: ARTERIAL AND VENOUS
   CLOTS   THROMBOSIS
   ↑PTT/↑PTT ∓ CORRECTION

DX: ANTI-CARDIOLIPIN (VDRL)
   LUPUS ANTI-COAGULANT
   B₂-GLYCOPROTEIN
   RUSSEL VIPER VENOM

TX: WARFARIN → ASA, LMWH

Musculoskeletal

Introduction to Skin

LAYERS OF SKIN

EPIDERMIS

DERMIS

SUB Q FAT — HYPODERMIS

FASCIA

STRATA EPIDERMIS

DESQUAMATION
CORNEUM—CORNEOCYTE

LUCIDUM

GRANULOSUM
- KERATOHYALINE GRANULES
- NUCLEAR DEGRADED

SPINOSUM
- NUCLEUS
- METABOLICALLY ACTIVE
- ORGANELLES

BASALE
- UNDIFFERENTIATED KERATINOCYTES
- STEM CELLS

DESCRIBING GROSS

COLOR	RAISED	FLUID—FILLED
< 1 CM	MACULE	PAPULE	VESICLES
> 1 CM	PATCH	NODULE (ROUND) PLAQUES (FLAT)	BULLA(E)

REMOVAL
EROSION — ULCER
FISSURE

DESCRIBE HISTOLOGY

C HYPERKERATOSIS – BIGGER CORNEUM
PARAKERATOSIS – NUCLEI IN CORNEUM

G HYPERGRANULOSIS – BIGGER GRANULOSUM

S SPONGIOSIS – FLUID/EDEMA
ACANTHOLYSIS – SEPARATION OF KERATINOCYTES

RETE RIDGE

PAPILLAE

CELLS OF EPIDERMIS

CORNEOCYTES = TERMINAL DIFFERENTIATION
KERATINOCYTES = KERATIN, SOFT
KERATOHYALINE GRANULES
DESMOSOMES MITOCHONDRIA
SQUAMOUS CELL CARCINOMA

BASAL CELLS = BM, HEMIDESMOSOMES
STEM CELL
CUBOID/COLUMNAR
BASAL CELL CARCINOMA

MELANOCYTE NEURAL CREST
PIGMENT
NEVI = MOLES
MELANOMA

CONNECTIONS

KERATINOCYTE   MELANOCYTES
DESMOSOMES   MELANOSOMES
DESMOGLEIN
DESMOPLAKIN

HEMIDESMOSOMES

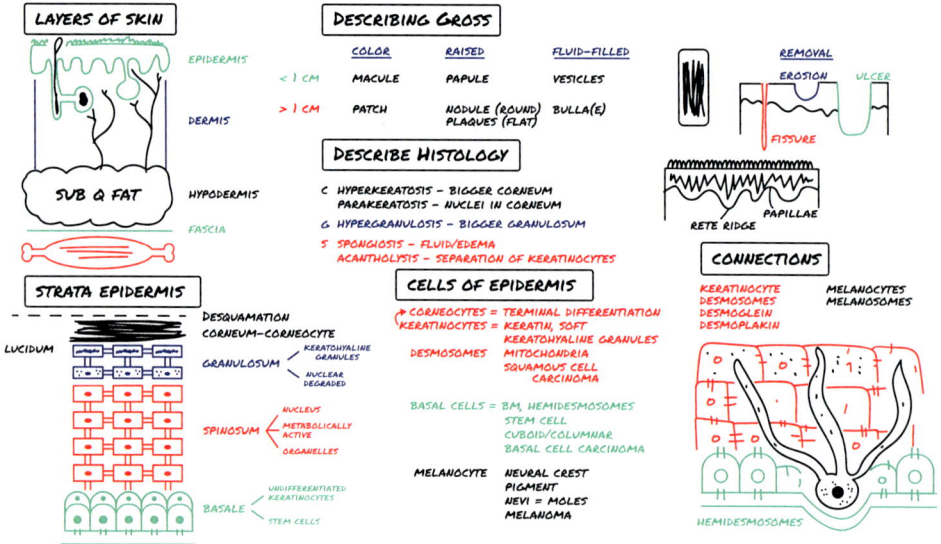

Disorders of Skin Pigmentation

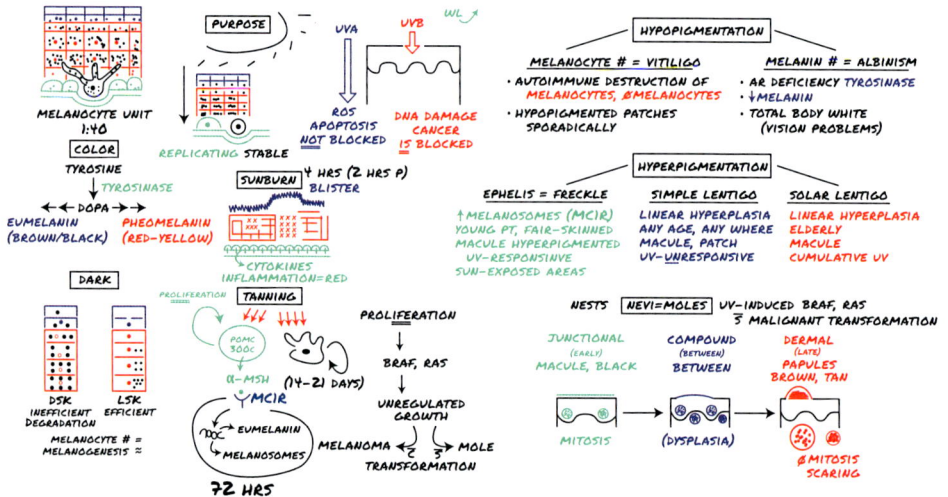

MELANOCYTE UNIT
1:40

COLOR
TYROSINE
↓ TYROSINASE
←← DOPA →→
EUMELANIN   PHEOMELANIN
(BROWN/BLACK)   (RED—YELLOW)

DARK

DSK   LSK
INEFFICIENT   EFFICIENT
DEGRADATION
MELANOCYTE # =
MELANOGENESIS ≈

PURPOSE

UVA   UVB   WL

ROS   DNA DAMAGE
APOPTOSIS   CANCER
NOT BLOCKED IS BLOCKED

REPLICATING STABLE

SUNBURN 4 HRS (2 HRS P) BLISTER

↑ CYTOKINES
INFLAMMATION=RED

PROLIFERATION

TANNING

POMC 300C
α—MSH (14–21 DAYS)
Ψ MCIR
DOC EUMELANIN
MELANOSOMES

72 HRS

PROLIFERATION
↓
BRAF, RAS
↓
UNREGULATED GROWTH
↓
MELANOMA ⇄ MOLE TRANSFORMATION

HYPOPIGMENTATION

MELANOCYTE # = VITILIGO
- AUTOIMMUNE DESTRUCTION OF MELANOCYTES, Ø MELANOCYTES
- HYPOPIGMENTED PATCHES SPORADICALLY

MELANIN # = ALBINISM
- AR DEFICIENCY TYROSINASE
- ↓ MELANIN
- TOTAL BODY WHITE (VISION PROBLEMS)

HYPERPIGMENTATION

EPHELIS = FRECKLE	SIMPLE LENTIGO (EARLY)	SOLAR LENTIGO
↑ MELANOSOMES (MC1R) YOUNG PT, FAIR—SKINNED MACULE HYPERPIGMENTED UV—RESPONSIVE SUN—EXPOSED AREAS	LINEAR HYPERPLASIA ANY AGE, ANY WHERE MACULE, PATCH UV—UNRESPONSIVE	LINEAR HYPERPLASIA ELDERLY MACULE CUMULATIVE UV

NESTS NEVI=MOLES UV-INDUCED BRAF, RAS
3 MALIGNANT TRANSFORMATION

JUNCTIONAL	COMPOUND (BETWEEN)	DERMAL (LATE)
MACULE, BLACK	BETWEEN	PAPULES BROWN, TAN
MITOSIS →	(DYSPLASIA) →	Ø MITOSIS SCARING

Musculoskeletal

Skin Cancers

SUN-EXPOSURE (BURN)
SUN-EXPOSED AREAS
SUN-OCCUPATION
SUN-BATHE

RTK = KIT → PI3K → AKT → MTOR → ANTI-APOPTOSIS
→ BRAF → CDK → PROLIFERATION

DOES WHAT MELANOCYTES DO = NESTS, PIGMENT

A SYMMETRY
B ORDER IRREGULARITIES
C OLOR VARIATION
D IAMETER > 1 CM
E VOLUTION

NESTS IN DERMIS S100⊕
MITOTICALLY ACTIVE
LARGE, MELANOCYTES LARGE
DYSPLASTIC NUCLEI

MELANOMA
MOST
DEADLY

BRAF ∅ ⊕

MOLES

BRAF-I = VEMURAFENIB

SK
NOT (PRE)MALIGNANT
UV EXPOSURE
ELDERLY "STUCK ON"
EPIDERMAL HYPERPLASIA
HYALINE PSEUDOCYSTS

ACTINIC KERATOSIS
PREMALIGNANT SCC
DIFFERENTIATED KERATINOCYTES
HYPERKERATOSIS HYPERPLASIA
PARAKERATOSIS
ERYTHEMATOUS PATCH, HORN

KERATOACANTHOMA
OBVIOUSLY SCC
RESOLVES SPONTANEOUSLY

XERODERMA PIGMENTOSUM
NER, P53
T-DIMERS

STEM CELL

SQUAMOUS CELL
CARCINOMA
(2ND MC CANCER)

DOES WHAT KERATINOCYTES DO
SUN CANCER, HPV, MARJOLIN ULCER
KERATIN WHORLS
DYSPLASTIC HYPERPLASIA
55

ERYTHEMATOUS, INDURATED, SCALING
NODULE, MAY ULCERATION
BOTTOM LIP

SONIC HEDGEHOG

BASAL CELL
CARCINOMA
(MC CANCER)

DOES WHAT BASAL CELLS DO
SUN CANCER
LEAST LIKELY TO METASTASIZE
LOCAL INVASION, AGGRESSIVE

UPPER LIP

BASOPHILIC BASALOID
ISLAND
PALLASIDING NUCLEI

WAXY/PEARLY PAPULES → NODULES
TELANGIECTASIAS = ⊕ BLOOD VESSELS

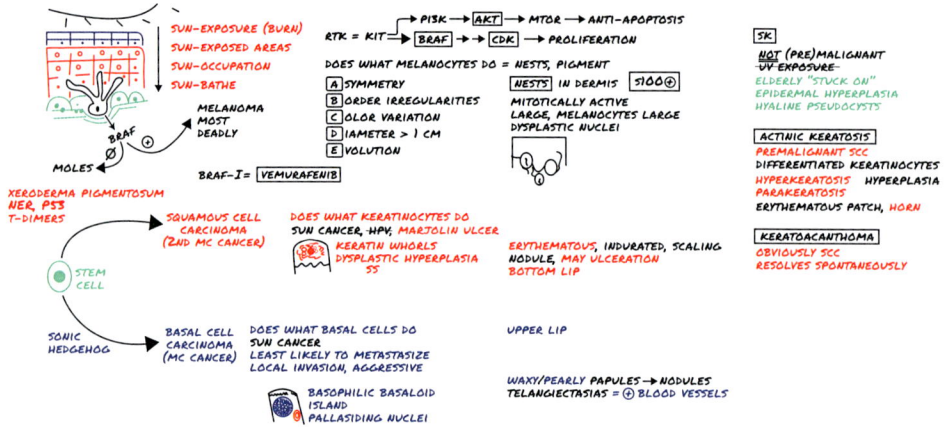

Blistering Diseases

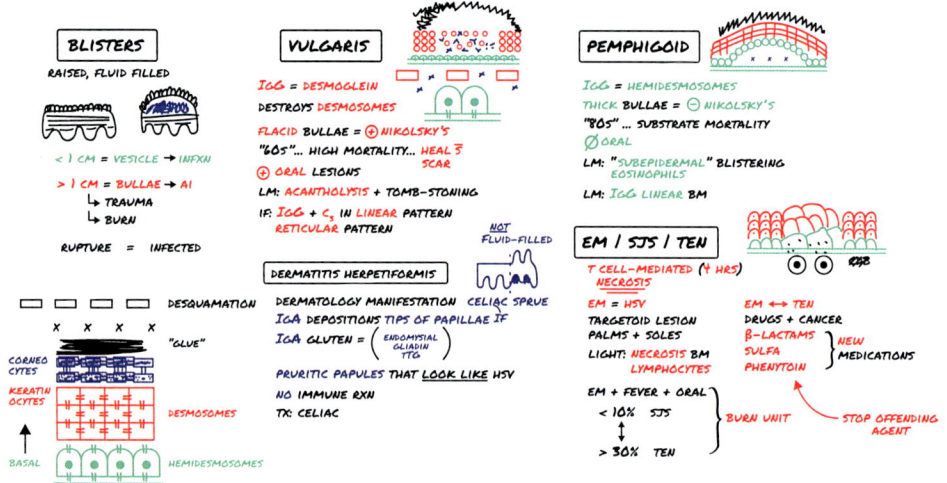

BLISTERS
RAISED, FLUID FILLED

< 1 CM = VESICLE → INFXN
> 1 CM = BULLAE → AI
  ↳ TRAUMA
  ↳ BURN
RUPTURE = INFECTED

DESQUAMATION

"GLUE"

CORNEO CYTES
KERATIN OCYTES
DESMOSOMES
BASAL
HEMIDESMOSOMES

VULGARIS
IGG = DESMOGLEIN
DESTROYS DESMOSOMES
FLACID BULLAE = ⊕ NIKOLSKY'S
"60S"... HIGH MORTALITY... HEAL 3̄
⊕ ORAL LESIONS SCAR
LM: ACANTHOLYSIS + TOMB-STONING
IF: IGG + C₃ IN LINEAR PATTERN
RETICULAR PATTERN

NOT FLUID-FILLED

DERMATITIS HERPETIFORMIS
DERMATOLOGY MANIFESTATION CELIAC SPRUE
IGA DEPOSITIONS TIPS OF PAPILLAE IF
IGA GLUTEN = (ENDOMYSIAL / GLIADIN / TTG)
PRURITIC PAPULES THAT LOOK LIKE HSV
NO IMMUNE RXN
TX: CELIAC

PEMPHIGOID
IGG = HEMIDESMOSOMES
THICK BULLAE = ⊖ NIKOLSKY'S
"80S" ... SUBSTRATE MORTALITY
∅ ORAL
LM: "SUBEPIDERMAL" BLISTERING
     EOSINOPHILS
LM: IGG LINEAR BM

EM / SJS / TEN
T CELL-MEDIATED (4 HRS)
NECROSIS
EM = HSV
TARGETOID LESION
PALMS + SOLES
LIGHT: NECROSIS BM
       LYMPHOCYTES
EM + FEVER + ORAL
< 10% SJS
> 30% TEN

EM ↔ TEN
DRUGS + CANCER
β-LACTAMS
SULFA   NEW
PHENYTOIN   MEDICATIONS

BURN UNIT
STOP OFFENDING AGENT

NOTES

Skin and Soft Tissue Infections

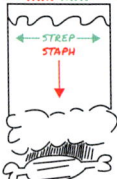

STAPH. AUREUS   GROUP A STREP. PYOGENES

← STREP →
STAPH

GROUP A STREP. PYOGENES — β-LACTAM
                         CEPHALOSPORIN
STAPH. AUREUS   — CEPHALOSPORIN
                 (MRSP) VANCOMYCIN

INFECTIONS

↑TEMP ↑WBC } SEPSIS
↑HR   ↑RR

SEVERITY SEPSIS
→ LOCATION OF TX
→ IV OR PO-ABX

IMPETIGO = EPIDERMIS
GROUP A STREP. PYOGENES
STAPH. AUREUS (BULLOUS) EXFOLATIN
KIDS, FACE, PUSTULES ERUPT
 COALESCE, HONEY-COLORED CRUST
UNTREATED → PSGN -RHEUMATIC♡

ERYSIPELAS DERMIS/EPIDERMIS
GROUP A STREP. PYOGENES
NORMAL → ANGRY FAST
SHARPLY-DEMARCATED = RED, HOT, TENDER
IF ON FACE, ∅ SPARE NLF

CELLULITIS SUB Q
INNOCULATION/PENETRATION TO SUB Q
 SPREADS OUT W/I SUB Q.
GROUP A STREP. OR STAPH. AUREUS
  PYOGENES   (BULLAE)
INSIDOUS ERYSIPELAS
NOT-DEMARCATED

NEC FAC
GROUP A STREP. PYOGENES
SAS — PURPLE/BLACK
   — POOP
BULLAE GAS = CREPITUS
SURGICAL EMERGENCY

OSTEOMYELITIS
① RECURRENT CELLULITIS
② SEPSIS + BONE PAIN
③ PROBE TO BONE   DX: X-RAY
MC: STAPH. AUREUS   MRI
SCD: SALMONELLA   BMBX
DM: PSEUDOMONAS TRACK: ESR+CRP
SNEAKER   TX: 6 WEEKS

ABSCESS
STAPH. AUREUS "ALWAYS"
WALLED OFF INFXN = ORGANISMS
FLUCTUANCE → I+D   PMN
        ↓
        → SPONTANEOUS → PUS

HAIR
 | MULTIPLE
FURUNCLE CARBUNCLE

Inflammatory Dermatoses

URTICARIA
WHEAL
EDEMA IN DERMIS
IgE-MAST CELL TYPE 1 HSR

ECZEMA { INSIDE = INGESTION
            OUTSIDE = APPLICATION
SCALING PLAQUE OOZES
ERYTHEMATOUS BASE

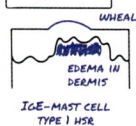
PARAKERATOSIS
HYPERKERATOSIS
SPONGIOSUS SS

① KID, NEW FOODS,   CD4 T   < 24 H: ERYTHEMA
   FACE, EXTENSORS HELPER   PRURITIS
② ADULT; FLEXORS (AC) CELLS > 24 H: PLAQUE
   CONTACT   INDUCED
                   PROLIFERATION

PSORIASIS

ELONGATED RETE: PROLIFERATION
ELONGATED PAPILLAE: CAPILLARIES
PT: ADULTS, SCALP, EXTENSORS
SILVER SCALING PLAQUES
ERYTHEMATOUS BASE
BLEED WHEN PICKED
NAIL PITTING
ONYCHOLYSIS

HISTO:
PARAKERATOSIS
HYPERKERATOSIS

THINNED EPIDERMIS (PAPILLAE)
UNIFORM ELONGATION RETE
ABSENT GRANULOSUM
NEUTROPHILS — MICROABSCESSES

TRUE ABSCESSES
(PUSTULAR)

SEBORRHEIC DERMATITIS
PATH: MALASSEZIA INFXN EPIDERMIS
      IDIOPATHIC INFLAMMATORY
      SEBACEOUS GLANDS, FOLLICLE
      HAIR IS THICK

PT: ① INFANTS = CRADLE CAP
    ② ADULTS = DANDRUFF
    YELLOW SCALING PLAQUE
    ERYTHEMATOUS BASE

HISTO:
PARAKERATOSIS
HYPERKERATOSIS
SPONGIOSUS

— — —

NEUTROPHILS —

TX: SELENIUM SHAMPOO
    TOPICAL ANTIFUNGAL
    IMMUNE MODULATORS

LICHEN PLANUS
PATH: ? HEP C ?

PT: Pruritic
    Pink / Purple
    Polygonal
    Planar
    Plaques

WICKHAM'S STRIAE
HISTO: HYPERGRANULOSIS

ERYTHEMA NODOSUM
RED TENDER NOD/PAPULE
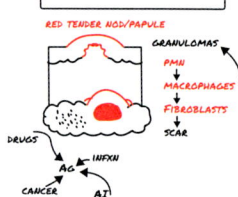
                    GRANULOMAS
                    PMN
                    MACROPHAGES
                    FIBROBLASTS
                    SCAR
DRUGS
        AG → INFXN
CANCER   AI

Musculoskeletal

Appendages of Skin

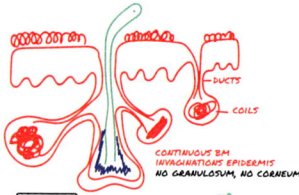

DUCTS

COILS

CONTINUOUS BM
INVAGINATIONS EPIDERMIS
NO GRANULOSUM, NO CORNEUM

SWEAT GLANDS

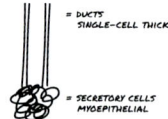

= DUCTS
SINGLE-CELL THICK

= SECRETORY CELLS
MYOEPITHELIAL

APOCRINE DEODORANT

HAIR FOLLICLE
FEW, LARGE
ANOGENITAL REGION
AXILLA

PHEROMONES, BACTERIA
EAT THEM → SMELL

ECCRINE ANTIPERSPIRANT

Ø HAIR FOLLICLE
EVERYWHERE, MANY
REGULATE TEMPERATURE

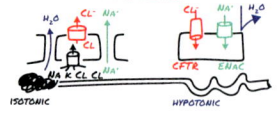

H_2O Cl^- Na^+ Cl^- Na^+ H_2O

Na^+ K^+ Cl^- Cl^- Na^+ CFTR   ENaC

ISOTONIC   HYPOTONIC

HAIR

BM = GLASSY

OUTER SHEATH
(EPIDERMIS)

INNER SHEATH
(HAIR FOLLICLE)

CUTICLE

CUTICLE

DP
CAPILLARY

MATRIX
(MELANOCYTES)

CORTEX
CORNEOCYTES
HARD KERATIN (S)
DON'T DESQUAMATE

INFUNDIBULUM

ISTHMUS

FOLLICULAR
BULGE

BULB

NAILS

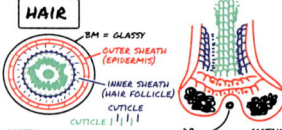
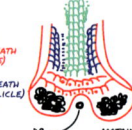

EPONYCHIUM

NAIL
PLATE

DORSAL

HYPO-
NYCHIUM

VENTRAL

NAIL BED

FOLLICLE	SHAFT
ANAGEN – PRO PROLIFERATE	PROLIFERATE
–META RESTS ANAGEN	PROLIFERATE
TELOGEN APOPTOSIS	PROLIFERATE
CATAGEN REST CATAGEN	STOPS

SEBACEOUS GLANDS

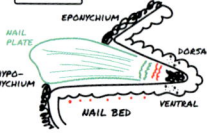

LIPID–LADEN
"CORNEOCYTES"
SEBUM

P. ACNE'S
INFLAMMATORY
FATTY ACIDS

OXIDIZED   Ø OXIDIZED

BLACKHEADS
CLOSED
COMEDONE

WHITEHEAD
OPEN
COMEDONE

ANDROGENS

↑ SEBUM

↑ BLOCKAGE

↑ P. ACNE

↑ FATTY ACIDS

PUSTULAR
COMEDONE

Musculoskeletal

The Healthy Esophagus

ANATOMY + VASCULATURE

INFERIOR THYROIDAL	SKEL MUSCLE	INFERIOR THYROIDAL
AZYGOS HEMIAZYGOS	TRANSITION	BRONCHIAL
INF VENA CAVA	SMOOTH MUSCLE	AORTA

UES

AORTA ANTERIOR UPPER MEDIASTINUM

AORTA POSTERIOR POSTERIOR MEDIASTINUM

T_{10}

LES

PORTAL VEIN

CELIAC

HISTOLOGY + LAYERS

EPITHELIUM
LAMINA PROPRIA
MUSCULARIS MUCOSA — MUCOSA

SUBMUCOSAL GLANDS
SUBMUCOSAL PLEXUS — SUBMUCOSA

CIRCULAR
LONGITUDINAL — MUSCULARIS EXTERNA

ADVENTITIA
MESOTHELIUM — SEROSA

MYENTERIC PLEXUS MOTILITY

PERITONEAL CAVITY

ESOPHAGEAL PHASE

↳ 1° PERISTALSIS
VAGUS-DEPENDENT
PHARYNGEAL INITIATED
① BEHIND = CONTRACTION → ACH
G_Q-IP3-Ca^{2+}
② FRONT = DILATION → NO → cGMP → RELAXATION
GTP
③ LES → NO, VIP

↳ 2° PERISTALSIS
VAGUS-INDEPENDENT
MYENTERIC PLEXUS COORDINATED
ETC

↳ NEUROTRANSMITTERS

ACH
VAGUS
2ND
ACH → CONTRACTION
NO → RED
2ND
VIP

GANGLION   W/ MYENTERIC PLEXUS

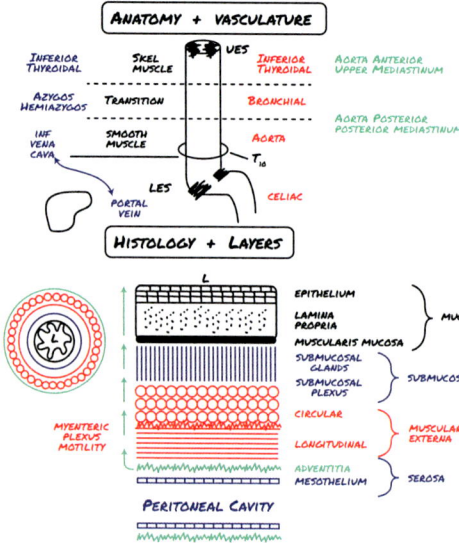

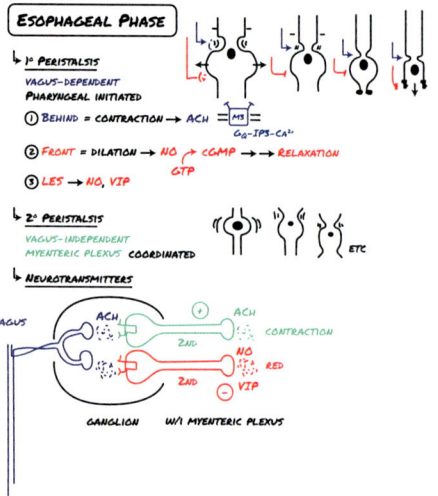

Esophageal Pathology

ANATOMIC PATH (EMESIS)

VARICES = PORTACAVAL SHUNT

LOWER ESOPHAGUS → PORTAL
UPPER ESOPHAGUS → CAVAL
CIRRHOTIC → PORTAL HTN
↳ ASX SCREEN... BB
↳ HEMATEMESIS... (ETOH)

MALLORY - WEISS

SUPERFICIAL LACERATION OF MUCOSA
"WEEKEND WARRIOR"... BINGE
VOMIT, VOMIT, VOMIT BLOOD,
VOMIT, VOMIT
SELF-LIMITING BLEED

BOERHAAVE'S SYNDROME

TRANSMURAL PERFORATION
"CAREER ALCOHOLIC"... BAD BINGE
(ETOH)... IATROGENIC

MEDIASTINITIS = TOXIC
↳ NO BLEEDING
↳ SUBQ EMPHYSEMA
↳ HAMMOND'S CRUNCH
↳ XRAY = AIR IN MEDIASTINUM

SURGICAL EMERGENCY

FUNCTIONAL PATH (DYSPHAGIA)

ACHALASIA

LOSS OF MYENTERIC PLEXUS

CHAGAS   1°   PSEUDO

-IMPAIRMENT LES OF RELAXATION
-IMPAIRMENT OF PERISTALSIS
-DYSPHAGIA TO FOOD + LIQUID
-BARIUM = BIRD'S BEAK
-MANOMETRY

[NUTCRACKER = DES] HTN

• UNCOORDINATED AND SIMULTANEOUS
  CONTRACTION
• SUBSTERNAL CP RELIEVED Ξ̄ NTG
  X̄ Ξ̄ CAD RF, EXACERBATED BY TEMP
• R/O ACS... R/O CAD
• BARIUM = NORMAL → CORKSCREW
  NITRATES OR CCB + NTG PRN

L_SS_ = CREST

• SMOOTH MUSCLE → COLLAGEN
  ↳ LES FAILS OF CONTRACT
  ↳ REFRACTORY GERD
• BARIUM = REFLUX
• MANOMETRY = LES Ξ̄ CONTRACTION

ANATOMIC PATH (CANCER)

SCC OF ESOPHAGUS

• ↑ 1/3 ESOPHAGUS
• SEMEN CAN GO... HPV CAN TOO
  HOT TEAS... POVERTY, ETOH, TOBACCO
• BARIUM: ECCENTRIC PROXIMAL
• NK STRATIFIED SQUAMOUS

GERD

• WEAKENED LES → H⁺ REFLUX
• HIATAL HERNIA, LCSS, HABITUS
• ETOH, TOBACCO, CHOCOLATE
• RETROSTERNAL BURNING CP
• WORSE Ξ̄ FLAT, IMPROVED ANTACIDS
• METALLIC TASTE, NOCTURNAL ASTHMA
• EGD WARNING SXS: EMESIS,
  ANEMIA, WEIGHT LOSS, OR
  FAILURE OF PPI X 6WEEKS

BARRETT'S

SALMON-COLORED ON BX
SIMPLE COLUMNAR EPITHELIUM
GERD RESOLVED SPONTANEOUSLY

ADENOCARCINOMA

• ↓ 1/3 ESOPHAGUS
GERD → INTESTINAL
       METAPLASIA
"GLANDS"
SIMPLE COLUMNAR
INVAGINATES
BARIUM → ECCENTRIC DISTAL

ESOPHAGITIS

PILL-INDUCED

INFECTIOUS
↳ HSV = (VAL)ACYCLOVIR
  PUNCHED-OUT, VESICLES
  MULTI-NUCLEATED GIANT CELLS

↳ CMV = (VAL)GANCICLOVIR
  LINEAR ULCER
  OWL'S EYES   PROFOUND

↳ CANDIDA = PO FLUCONAZOLE
  ADHERENT WHITE   AIDS
  PSEUDOHYPHAE

EOSINOPHILIC
• ≥ 15 EOS/HPF + FAILURE OF GERD
• ASTHMA ALLERGIES ATOPY
• PO INH STEROIDS
• RINGS

CAUSTIC

GERD

62

© 2021 OnlineMedEd

NOTES

Anatomy and Histology of the Stomach

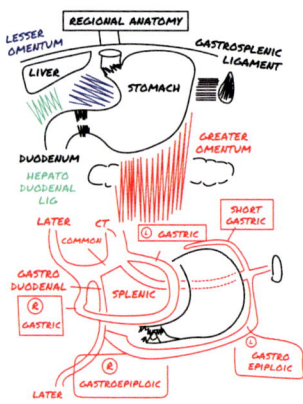

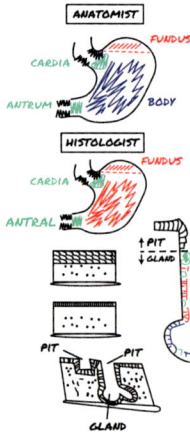

REGIONAL ANATOMY

LESSER OMENTUM
LIVER
GASTROSPLENIC LIGAMENT
STOMACH
DUODENUM
GREATER OMENTUM
HEPATO DUODENAL LIG
SHORT GASTRIC
LATER CT
COMMON
L GASTRIC
GASTRO DUODENAL
SPLENIC
R GASTRIC
GASTRO EPIPLOIC
R GASTROEPIPLOIC
LATER

ANATOMIST

FUNDUS
CARDIA
ANTRUM
BODY

HISTOLOGIST

FUNDUS
CARDIA
ANTRAL

↑ PIT
↓ GLAND
ISTHMUS
NECK
FUNDUS
HISTAMINE
PIT
PIT
GLAND

MECHANICAL DIGESTION

① CHURNING (OBLIQUE) MULLING OVER
② PROPULSION, RETROPULSION PERISTALSIS SLAMS INTO PYLORUS = PULVERIZING
③ GRINDING SUPER CHURN

CELLS OF STOMACH

MUCOSAL = MUCUS, BICARB GEL-LIKE COAT SURFACE, PITS

STEM CELLS = PIT/SURFACE GLANDS

PARIETAL CELLS = H⁺ → HCl = IF

CHIEF CELLS = PEPSINOGEN

ECL CELLS = HISTAMINE ENDOCRINE, "PARACRINE"

ANTRUM
└ G CELLS = GASTRIN

Physiology and Pharmacology of the Stomach

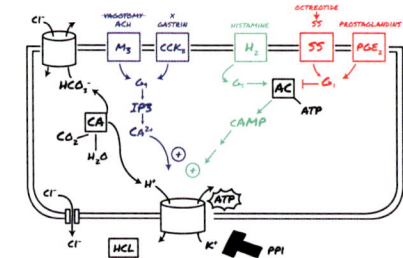

VAGOTOMY ACH
X GASTRIN
HISTAMINE
OCTREOTIDE
SS PROSTAGLANDINS
PROSTAGLANDINS NSAID, ASA
MISOPROSTOL

Cl⁻
M_3 CCK_B H_2 SS PGE_2
HCO₃⁻ Gq
CA IP3 Gi AC Gs
CO₂ CA²⁺ CAMP ATP
H₂O H⁺
Cl⁻ ATP
Cl⁻ K⁺ PPI
HCL

PHASES OF EATING

① CEPHALIC PHASE = "PREP PHASE"
② GASTRIC PHASE = INITIATING DIGESTION H⁺, PEPSIN... PROPULSION, CHURNING, GRINDING
③ INTESTINAL PHASE = TERMINAL DIGESTION + ABSORPTION D, S, I, K

PHARMACOLOGY

OK ① PROTON PUMP INHIBITORS
  - IRREVERSIBLY INHIBIT H⁺-K⁺ATPase
  - SLOW TO EFFECT
  - TX : PUD, GERD, BARRETT'S
  - SE : ↑ GASTRIN (100), ↓ K, ↓ CA ⟹ OSTEOPOROSIS, C. DIFF, PNA
  + STRESS ULCER PPX ⟹ NNN (C. DIFF) < NNT (ULCERS)
    └ NOW IN THE ICU

② H₂ BLOCKERS - TIDINE RANITIDINE, FAMOTIDINE, CIMETIDINE
  └ FASTER ACTING, BID

---

③ ANTACIDS = SUPER FAST ACTING, RAPID RELIEF USEFUL FOR DX THAN TX

④ BISMUTH   SUCRALFATE = "COATING"
  └ STOOL BLACK   └ NOT ABSORBED └ PUD, GERD

SIGNALING TOO HARD!

VAGOTOMY ACH
LAMA = COPD COPD
GASTRIN

OCTREOTIDE SS
(ZOLLINGER-ELLISON)
PROSTAGLANDIN

WARFARIN TOXICITY
├ P450-, -
├ PGP
└ ANTI-ANDROGENS

CELL	STIMULATED BY	MAKES	INHIBITED BY	PARIETAL PRODUCTION
ECL (GLANDS)	ACH GASTRIN	HISTAMINES	SS	↑
G CELLS (ANTRUM)	AA-Trp PHE GRP (ACH)	GASTRIN	SS	↑
D CELLS (DUODENUM)	GASTRIN H⁺	SOMATOSTATIN (SS)	ACH	↓
VAGUS (NEUROTRANSMITTERS)	CEPHALIC PHASE GASTRIC DISTENTION	ACH GRP	–	↑

Gastrointestinal

Gastric Pathology

ACUTE GASTRITIS

⬇ = NSAIDS, ETOH, TOBACCO, H.PYLORI

MUCUS
PERI-
CILIARY
LAYER

ALKALINE TIDE
O_2 → GLUCOSE ⊢ ISCHEMIA
PROSTAGLANDINS ⊢ NSAIDS

GASTRITIS = IMMUNE CELLS ⊃ EROSION
EROSION = INTO MUCOSA, ABOVE MM
ULCER = THROUGH MUCOSA, INTO SUB

ACUTE ULCERS

CUSHING'S = ↑ICP

⬆ BP ⬇ HR

CURLING'S = BURN

W/O BURN, IN BURN UNIT
STRESS ULCER = SEVERE DZ — PPX
ICU, INTUBATED, PRESSORS
NNT << NNH
75% ICU = STRESS ULCER
FEEDING > H_2 BLOCKERS > PPI

CHRONIC GASTRITIS

SXS : DYSPEPSIA : BLOATED
BELCHING, EARLY SATIETY,
NAUSEA, WEIGHT LOSS

PERNICIOUS ANEMIA = TYPE 2 HSR
ANTIPARIETAL   ANTIIF   ANTI-PP

⊢ GASTRIC ATROPHY + ⬇B_{12} DEFICIENCY

(↑HCL) ACHLORHYDRIA   MACROCYTIC ANEMIA
                        NEUROLOGIC SXS

↑GASTRIN   ↑ADENOCARCINOMA

⊢ CARCINOID

H/O ANOTHER AI DISEASE
                        MALTOMA

H. PYLORI INFXN | ADENOCARCINOMA

TREATING AN INFXN PREVENTS CANCER
UREASE (↑PH) ANTRUM (NON FUNDUS)
EGD ⊃ BX
⊢ GRAM ⊖ RODS
⊢ INTRAEPITHELIAL PMN
⊢ PLASMA CELLS IN CD

SEROLOGY   T+T STRATEGY
UREA BREATH TEST   CONFIRM REINFECTION
STOOL AG   CONFIRMS ERADICATION
EGD ⊃ BX   BEST OVERALL, RITH

"OTHER" CHRONIC GASTRITIS

ETOH   TOBACCO   NSAIDS

↑ RISK   CAUSE

PEPTIC ULCER DZ

SXS : GNAWING EPIGASTRIC PAIN
BORES TO BACK △S ⊃ FOOD

① GASTRIC ULCERS
"WORST" ⊃ FOOD
EGD - APPEARANCE
⊢ MULTIPLE, SMALL   NSAIDS
⊢ SHARP, LARGE   STRESS
⊢ HEAPED, LARGE   CANCER
  UP
⊢ SINGULAR, LARGE   H.PYLORI
⊢ MULTIPLE, LARGE   ZE

② DUODENAL ULCER
"IMPROVE" ⊃ FOOD
≈ 100% H. PYLORI (ZE)
≈ 100% PROXIMAL (TEST)
        DUODENUM
H.PYLORI...BRUNNER'S

③ ZOLLINGER - ELLISON
(1000S) GASTRIN SECRETING
PANCREATIC NEOPLASM
MULTIPLE, LARGE, REFRACTORY ULCERS
⇧ MALIGNANT TRANSFORMATION
   STOMACH CANCER

ADENOCARCINOMA

PATH : H. PYLORI   NITROSAMINE
       (ABX)   (UNUSED)

INCIDENCE ↓↓↓
SCREENING ↓⊃   EGD

WEIRD STUFF VIRCHOW'S NODE: SUPRACLAVICULAR
(TEST) SISTER MARY JOSEPH NODULE : UMBILICAL
       KRUKENBERG TUMOR : OVARY
       POOR PROGNOSIS... EARLY SATIETY

HISTOLOGY

INTESTINAL TYPE
⊢ H. PYLORI + INTESTINAL METAPLASIC
⊢ GENETICS β-CATENIN

DIFFUSE TYPE
⊢ SIGNET RING CELLS
⊢ LINITIS PLASTICA
⊢ GENETICS APC

Anatomy of the Digestive Unit

ANATOMY + VASCULATURE

HEAD PANCREAS TAIL

SMA

PANCREAS

CELIAC TRUNK → SPLENIC A → DORSAL
                            PANCREATIC

CHA → GASTRO- → SUP. PANCREATICO-
      DUODENAL   DUODENAL

SMA → INFERIOR PANCREATICODUODENAL

DUODENUM

↑1/3 CT → CHA → GASTRO- → SUP. PANCREATICO-
                 DUODENAL   DUODENAL

MID 1/3 SMA → INFERIOR PANCREATICODUODENAL

↓1/3 SMA → 1ST JEJUNAL

GUT EMBRYOLOGY VASCULATURE

FOREGUT = DIGESTION, CELIAC TRUNK
⊢ STOMACH, 1/3 DUODENUM, LIVER,
  PANCREAS, GALLBLADDER

MIDGUT = ABSORPTION, SMA
⊢ DISTAL 2/3 DUODENUM JEJUNUM
  ILEUM UP TO 1ST 2/3 TRANSVERSE COLON

HINDGUT = EXPULSION, IMA
  REST OF COLON RECTUM AND CANAL

PANCREATIC EMBRYO

DORSAL BUD = "PANCREAS" HEAD → TAIL
VENTRAL BUD = "AMPULLA OF VATER" HEAD, UNCINATE
DIVISIUM = FAILURE TO FUSE CBD, PANCREATIC
ANNULAR PANCREAS = 2 VENTRAL BUDS → RING

PANCREATIC HISTOLOGY

ACINAR CELLS = ACINUS
CLUSTER OF CELLS ⊃ SHARED LUMEN
ZYMOGENS VIA CCK

DUCTAL CELLS
LINE DUCTS + SECRETE BICARB AQUEOUS
SECRETIN (⊃ DUODENUM)

DUODENUM HISTOLOGY

HISTOLOGY

                        VILLI

                        "SURFACE"
                        CRYPT

EPITHELIUM = SIMPLE COLUMNAR
"GLANDS" = INTESTINAL CRYPTS
VILLI = EXTENSION FROM "SURFACE"
MICROVILLI = FINGERLIKE PROJECTIONS
             ON CELLS

CELLS + PHYSIOLOGY

GOBLET CELLS = "MUCOSAL"
WHITE, FILLED ⊃ LIPID
↑ # IN COLON

M CELLS = SAMPLERS
ENTIRE ANTIGENS, ORGANISMS

ENTEROCYTE = ABSORBER
TERMINAL DIGESTION
ABSORPTION + ENTEROENDOCRINE

∧ PANETH CELLS

▯ INTERMEDIATE CELL

⊙ STEM CELL

DUODENAL EMBRYO

① HOLLOW TUBE
② OVERPROLIFERATION
③ RECANALIZATION
④ FAILURE = ATRESIA

DOUBLE BUBBLE

ANNULAR   DUODENAL
PANCREAS   ATRESIA
             (TRISOMY)

+/- BILIOUS EMESIS

SOME AIR IN COLON
(PARTIAL)

∅ AIR IN COLON
(COMPLETE)

SURGERY

Gastrointestinal

Physiology of Digestion and Absorption

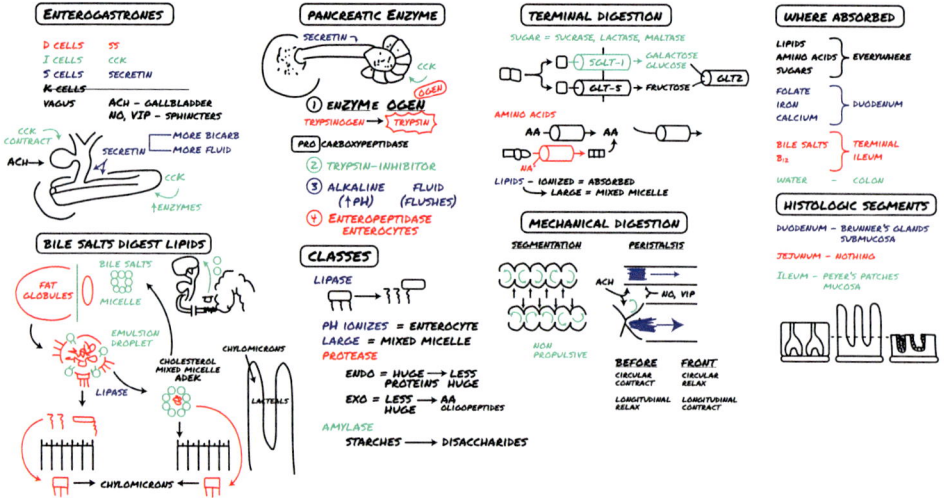

ENTEROGASTRONES

D CELLS	SS
I CELLS	CCK
S CELLS	SECRETIN
K CELLS	
VAGUS	ACH – GALLBLADDER
	NO, VIP – SPHINCTERS

CCK – CONTRACT
ACH
SECRETIN – MORE BICARB, MORE FLUID
CCK ↑ENZYMES

BILE SALTS DIGEST LIPIDS

FAT GLOBULES
BILE SALTS
MICELLE
EMULSION DROPLET
CHOLESTEROL MIXED MICELLE ADEK
LIPASE
CHYLOMICRONS
LACTEALS
CHYLOMICRONS

PANCREATIC ENZYME

SECRETIN
CCK
OGEN
① ENZYME OGEN
TRYPSINOGEN → TRYPSIN
PRO CARBOXYPEPTIDASE
② TRYPSIN–INHIBITOR
③ ALKALINE FLUID (↑PH) (FLUSHES)
④ ENTEROPEPTIDASE ENTEROCYTES

CLASSES

LIPASE
PH IONIZES = ENTEROCYTE
LARGE = MIXED MICELLE
PROTEASE
ENDO = HUGE → LESS PROTEINS HUGE
EXO = LESS → AA HUGE OLIGOPEPTIDES
AMYLASE
STARCHES → DISACCHARIDES

TERMINAL DIGESTION

SUGAR = SUCRASE, LACTASE, MALTASE
SGLT-1
GALACTOSE GLUCOSE
GLT-5 → FRUCTOSE
GLT2
AMINO ACIDS
AA → AA
Na
LIPIDS – IONIZED = ABSORBED
LARGE = MIXED MICELLE

MECHANICAL DIGESTION

SEGMENTATION   PERISTALSIS
ACH
NO, VIP
NON PROPULSIVE

BEFORE	FRONT
CIRCULAR CONTRACT	CIRCULAR RELAX
LONGITUDINAL RELAX	LONGITUDINAL CONTRACT

WHERE ABSORBED

LIPIDS, AMINO ACIDS, SUGARS – EVERYWHERE
FOLATE, IRON, CALCIUM – DUODENUM
BILE SALTS, B12 – TERMINAL ILEUM
WATER – COLON

HISTOLOGIC SEGMENTS

DUODENUM – BRUNNER'S GLANDS SUBMUCOSA
JEJUNUM – NOTHING
ILEUM – PEYER'S PATCHES MUCOSA

Malabsorption

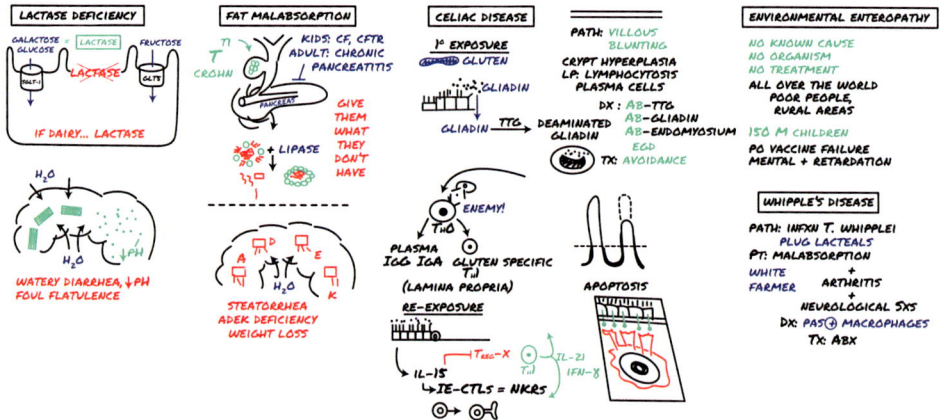

LACTASE DEFICIENCY

GALACTOSE GLUCOSE
LACTASE
FRUCTOSE
SGLT-1
GLTS
LACTASE
IF DAIRY... LACTASE
H_2O
H_2O
↓PH
WATERY DIARRHEA, ↓PH
FOUL FLATULENCE

FAT MALABSORPTION

TI
CROHN
KIDS: CF, CFTR
ADULT: CHRONIC PANCREATITIS
PANCREAT
LIPASE
GIVE THEM WHAT THEY DON'T HAVE
A D E K
H_2O
STEATORRHEA
ADEK DEFICIENCY
WEIGHT LOSS

CELIAC DISEASE

1° EXPOSURE
GLUTEN
GLIADIN
GLIADIN → TTG → DEAMINATED GLIADIN
ENEMY!
PLASMA IgG IgA GLUTEN SPECIFIC
(LAMINA PROPRIA)
RE-EXPOSURE
T_{REG}-X
IL-21
Th
IFN-γ
IL-15
IE-CTLs = NKRs

PATH: VILLOUS BLUNTING
CRYPT HYPERPLASIA
LP: LYMPHOCYTOSIS PLASMA CELLS
DX: AB-TTG
AB-GLIADIN
AB-ENDOMYOSIUM
EGD
TX: AVOIDANCE
APOPTOSIS

ENVIRONMENTAL ENTEROPATHY

NO KNOWN CAUSE
NO ORGANISM
NO TREATMENT
ALL OVER THE WORLD
POOR PEOPLE, RURAL AREAS
150 M CHILDREN
PO VACCINE FAILURE
MENTAL + RETARDATION

WHIPPLE'S DISEASE

PATH: INFXN T. WHIPPLEI PLUG LACTEALS
PT: MALABSORPTION + ARTHRITIS + NEUROLOGICAL SXS
WHITE FARMER
DX: PAS⊕ MACROPHAGES
TX: ABX

NOTES

Pancreatic Pathology

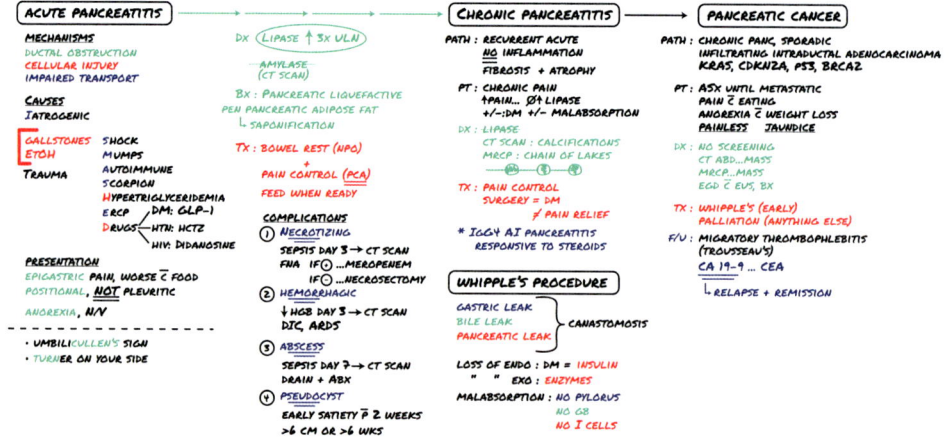

ACUTE PANCREATITIS

MECHANISMS
DUCTAL OBSTRUCTION
CELLULAR INJURY
IMPAIRED TRANSPORT

CAUSES
IATROGENIC

GALLSTONES   SHOCK
ETOH   MUMPS
TRAUMA   AUTOIMMUNE
            SCORPION
            HYPERTRIGLYCERIDEMIA
            ERCP ─ DM: GLP-1
            DRUGS ┬ HTN: HCTZ
                  └ HIV: DIDANOSINE

PRESENTATION
EPIGASTRIC PAIN, WORSE c̄ FOOD
POSITIONAL, **NOT** PLEURITIC

ANOREXIA, N/V
- - - - - - - - - - - - - - - - -
• UMBILI CULLEN'S SIGN
• TURNER ON YOUR SIDE

DX (LIPASE ↑ 3x ULN)
    ─ AMYLASE
      (CT SCAN)
BX : PANCREATIC LIQUEFACTIVE
     PEN PANCREATIC ADIPOSE FAT
     └ SAPONIFICATION

TX : BOWEL REST (NPO)
         +
     PAIN CONTROL (PCA)
     FEED WHEN READY

COMPLICATIONS
① NECROTIZING
   SEPSIS DAY 3 → CT SCAN
   FNA IF ⊕ ...MEROPENEM
        IF ⊖ ...NECROSECTOMY
② HEMORRHAGIC
   ↓ HGB DAY 3 → CT SCAN
   DIC, ARDS
③ ABSCESS
   SEPSIS DAY 7 → CT SCAN
   DRAIN + ABX
④ PSEUDOCYST
   EARLY SATIETY p̄ 2 WEEKS
   >6 CM OR >6 WKS

CHRONIC PANCREATITIS

PATH : RECURRENT ACUTE
       <u>NO</u> INFLAMMATION
       FIBROSIS + ATROPHY
PT : CHRONIC PAIN
     ↑PAIN... Ø↑ LIPASE
     +/−:DM +/− MALABSORPTION
DX : LIPASE
     CT SCAN : CALCIFICATIONS
     MRCP : CHAIN OF LAKES
     ─ ⊗ ─ ⊗ ─ ⊗ ─
TX : PAIN CONTROL
     SURGERY = DM
              ↓ PAIN RELIEF

* IgG4 AI PANCREATITIS
  RESPONSIVE TO STEROIDS

WHIPPLE'S PROCEDURE

GASTRIC LEAK
BILE LEAK   ─ CANASTOMOSIS
PANCREATIC LEAK

LOSS OF ENDO : DM = INSULIN
    "   "   : EXO = ENZYMES
MALABSORPTION : NO PYLORUS
                NO GB
                NO I CELLS

PANCREATIC CANCER

PATH : CHRONIC PANC, SPORADIC
       INFILTRATING INTRADUCTAL ADENOCARCINOMA
       KRAS, CDKN2A, p53, BRCA2
PT : ASX UNTIL METASTATIC
     PAIN c̄ EATING
     ANOREXIA c̄ WEIGHT LOSS
     PAINLESS JAUNDICE
DX : NO SCREENING
     CT ABD...MASS
     MRCP...MASS
     EGD c̄ EUS, BX
TX : WHIPPLE'S (EARLY)
     PALLIATION (ANYTHING ELSE)
F/U : MIGRATORY THROMBOPHLEBITIS
      (TROUSSEAU'S)
      CA 19-9 ... CEA
      └ RELAPSE + REMISSION

The Healthy Large Intestine

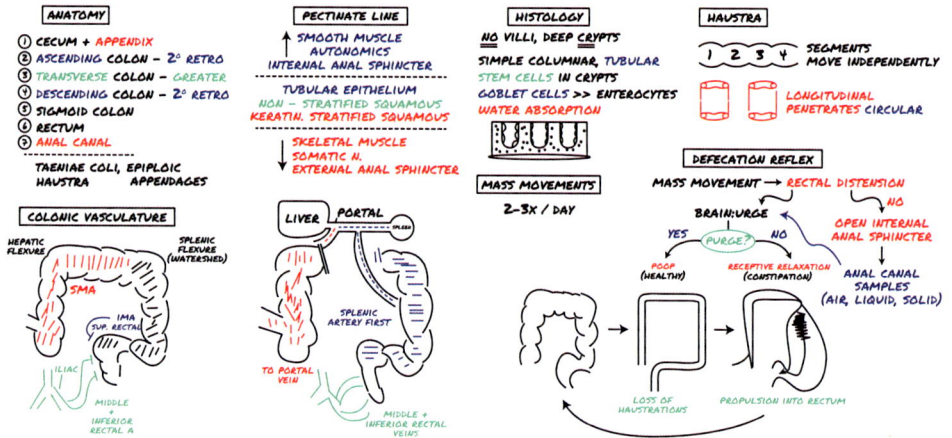

ANATOMY
① CECUM + APPENDIX
② ASCENDING COLON – 2° RETRO
③ TRANSVERSE COLON – GREATER
④ DESCENDING COLON – 2° RETRO
⑤ SIGMOID COLON
⑥ RECTUM
⑦ ANAL CANAL
- - - - - - - - - - - - - -
TAENIAE COLI, EPIPLOIC
HAUSTRA   APPENDAGES

COLONIC VASCULATURE
HEPATIC   SPLENIC
FLEXURE   FLEXURE
                 (WATERSHED)
        SMA
        IMA
        SUP. RECTAL
ILIAC
        MIDDLE
          +
        INFERIOR
        RECTAL A

PECTINATE LINE
↑ SMOOTH MUSCLE
  AUTONOMICS
  INTERNAL ANAL SPHINCTER
- - - - - - - - - - - - - - - -
  TUBULAR EPITHELIUM
NON – STRATIFIED SQUAMOUS
KERATIN. STRATIFIED SQUAMOUS
↓ SKELETAL MUSCLE
  SOMATIC N.
  EXTERNAL ANAL SPHINCTER

LIVER PORTAL
                 SPLEEN

              SPLENIC
              ARTERY FIRST
TO PORTAL
VEIN
              MIDDLE +
              INFERIOR RECTAL
              VEINS

HISTOLOGY
NO VILLI, DEEP CRYPTS
SIMPLE COLUMNAR, TUBULAR
STEM CELLS IN CRYPTS
GOBLET CELLS >> ENTEROCYTES
WATER ABSORPTION

MASS MOVEMENTS
2-3x / DAY

HAUSTRA
1 2 3 4   SEGMENTS
          MOVE INDEPENDENTLY

          LONGITUDINAL
          PENETRATES CIRCULAR

DEFECATION REFLEX
MASS MOVEMENT → RECTAL DISTENSION
                              NO
     BRAIN:URGE
YES   NO   OPEN INTERNAL
    (PURGE?)   ANAL SPHINCTER
POOP   RECEPTIVE RELAXATION   ANAL CANAL
(HEALTHY) (CONSTIPATION)   SAMPLES
                                 (AIR, LIQUID, SOLID)

LOSS OF   PROPULSION INTO RECTUM
HAUSTRATIONS

Gastrointestinal

Neoplasia of Large Intestine

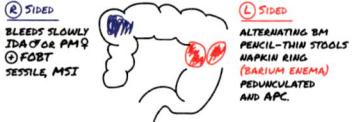

POLYPS

"REASSURING"
♀ SMALL <2 CM
PEDUNCULATED
TUBULAR HISTOLOGY

"NONREASSURING"
LARGE ≥ 2 CM
SESSILE
VILLOUS HISTOLOGY

POLYP = PREMALIGNANT
SCREENING WE __PREVENT__ CANCER

STAGE
MATTERS
MOST

OTHER POLYPS

HYPERPLASTIC (60-70)
ENDO = AD/CAR
HISTO = Ø

JUVENILE POLYPS
RICH LAMINA PROPRIA
"ARBORIZATION"

PEUTZ-JEGHERS
SI HAMARTOMATOUS POLYPS
MUCOCUTANEOUS PIGMENTS

ADENOMA-CARCINOMA

GENE	MUCOSA
APC	NORMAL
COX-2	HYPERPROLIFERATION (ASA CHEMOPROTECTIVE)
KRAS	PEDUNCULATED POLYP
P53	MALIGNANCY

"COLON CANCER" = ADENOMA CARCINOMA
PEDUNCULATED → CANCER
↳ MUCOSA → ADENOMA

FAP = APC DEF. __AD__
↳ 1000s POLYPS @18
↳ DEAD @30
↳ PPX COLECTOMY
FAP + OSTEOMAS = GARDENER'S
FAP + BRAIN = TURCOT'S TURBAN

MSI "PROGRESSION" ⟹ LYNCH ⟹ HNP CC

DNA MISMATCH REPAIR

GENE	MUCOSA
MLH1 OR MSH2	NORMAL
"2ND HIT"	PROLIFERATION
BAX	"
TGF-β-R	MALIGNANCY
BRAF	

3:2:1
1° RELATIVE, LYNCH
2° OVARIES
<50 COLON
PANCREAS

CLINICAL CRC + SCREENING

Ⓡ SIDED
BLEEDS SLOWLY
IDA ♂ OR PM ♀
⊕ FOBT
SESSILE, MSI

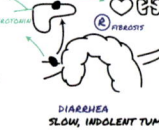

Ⓛ SIDED
ALTERNATING BM
PENCIL-THIN STOOLS
NAPKIN RING
(BARIUM ENEMA)
PEDUNCULATED
AND APC.

COLON CANCER SCREENING PREVENTS CA
* BEST = COLONOSCOPY
50 10 YRS W/I 1° 8 YR UC

ALTERNATE
FOBT q3Y
+
FLEXSIG q5Y

*CHEAP
FOBT q1Y
(FIT)

CARCINOID [FLUSHING]

SEROTONIN

Ⓡ FIBROSIS

DIARRHEA
SLOW, INDOLENT TUMORS   5-HIAA

ANAL CANCER
PATH : NK-SCC
SEMEN = HPV
PT : ANORECEPTIVE SEX
♀ >> ♂, MSM
DX : BX = NK-SCC
TX : EXQUISITELY SENSITIVE
TO CHEMO

Functional Intestinal Disease

TYPES OF DIARRHEA

	WBC/RBC	FASTING	OSMOLE GAP
SECRETORY	Ø	Ø	Ø
OSMOTIC (MALABSORPTION)	Ø	⊕△ (SLOW)	⊕
INFLAMMATORY INVASIVE	⊕	Ø	Ø

MEGACOLON

[TOXIC] MEGACOLON
ULCERATIVE COLITIS
C. DIFF COLITIS
DILATED BOWEL IS NORMAL

GOOD
BAD

[JUST] MEGACOLON
↳ HIRSCHSPRUNG'S (CONGENITAL)
- NEURAL CREST MIGRATION
NEO - DISTAL GUT TUBE
NODE - ↓TPM, INTACT ANUS,
- ABSENT MYENTERIC PLEXUS
↳ CHAGAS
ADULT T. CRUZI DESTROYS MYSTERIC
PLEXUS
(ESOPHAGUS, COLON, SI, UTERUS)
ENDEMIC

SECRETORY DIARRHEA

VIP-R   SEROTONIN
Gs   CAM   Gs
PKA   KINASE
ET ET PKG   Cl⁻

BISMUTH?

LOPERAMIDE DIPHENOXYLATE
OCTREOTIDE ADSORBENTS

CONSTIPATION = MOTILITY + SOFT STOOL

[LAXATIVES] ↗ ABUSE
① OSMOTIC MAGNESIUM
CIRRHOSIS — (LACTULOSE)
HE
② BULKING PSYLLIUM
METHYLCELLULOSE
③ LUBRICANT MINERAL OIL (PO)
GLYCERIN (PR)
④ MOTILITY [SENNA]
BISACODYL

[SOFTENERS]
DOCUSATE (PO)

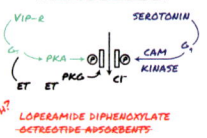

MASS MOVEMENT

DEFECATION

RECEPTIVE
RELAXATION

IMPACTION

SPECIFIC

OIC - METHYLNALTREXONE
OGILVIE'S - NEOSTIGMINE
REFRACTORY-LUBIPROSTONE

OSMOTIC DIARRHEA

FAT MALABSORPTION
ADEK
STEATORRHEA
CHRONIC/ORLISTAT

CARBOHYDRATE MAL
- LACTOSE, ↓STOOL PH
- CELIAC DISEASE
- LAXATIVES (MG)

ANTIEMETICS

[VESTIBULAR]   [CT2] ⊕   [GUT R]

M_1 = SCOPOLAMINE
H_1 = PROMETHAZINE

CHEMO
[CT2]
5-HT₃ ONDANSETRON
NK-1 APREPITANT

VOMITING
CENTER
INITIATES +
COORDINATES
EMESIS

[BRAIN/CORTEX]
D_2-MET
GABA - BENZOS (ADJUNCT)

?

STEROIDS
DEXAMETHASONE

INFILTRATIVE DIARRHEA

MEDICAL DZ (UC)

EHEC
SHIGELLA
SALMONELLA
YERSINIA

C. DIFF
AMOEBA HISTOLOGY
CAMPYLOBACTER
AEROMONAS

CALPROTECTIN (WBC)
LACTOFERRIN (RBC)

D_2 - METOCLOPRAMIDE
↓ NAUSEA
↑ GUT MOTILITY
GASTROPARESIS
EXTRA-PYRAMIDAL

Gastrointestinal

ULCERATIVE COLITIS

$T_H 17$ (PMNs)	MECH
CRYPT ABSCESS	HISTO
MUCOSA...SUBMUCOSA	DEPTH
BROAD-BASED	SHAPE
RECTUM → PROCTITIS	LOCATION
↓ COLITIS	
ENTIRE → PROCTITIS	
CONTINUOUS ULCER	ENDOSCOPY
SHARPLY DEMARCATED	
PSEUDOPOLYPS	
BLOODY, Ø△ WEIGHT	DIARRHEA
LEAD-PIPE SIGN	BARIUM
CURATIVE	SURGERY

Ø	FIBROSIS	⊕
Ø	FISTULA	⊕
Ø	STRICTURE	⊕
COLON CANCER @8 YEARS OF DX qIY	CANCER	↑COLON CA
PPX HEMICOLECTOMY PSC (ALP qIY)	EXTRA -😊	UVEITIS ARTHRITIS

CROHN'S DISEASE

$T_H 1$ (MACROPHAGES)	
NONCASEATING GRANULOMA	
TRANSMURAL	
KNIFE-LIKE	
ANYWHERE IN GI TRACT	
* TERMINAL ILEUM	
SKIP LESIONS + COBBLESTONING	
WATERY, ↓ WEIGHT	
STRING SIGN	
COMPLICATIONS	

MICROSCOPIC COLITIS

30-50 YO F c̄ DIARRHEA
REFRACTORY, ALL TESTS ⊖
COLONOSCOPY = NORMAL
HISTOLOGY = ABNORMAL

COLLAGENOUS   LYMPHOCYTIC

APPENDICITIS

PATH : APPENDIX = VESTIGIAL
FECALITH (ADULT)
LYMPHOID HYPERPLASIA (KIDS)
PT : PERIUMBILICAL PAIN
– MIGRATES TO MCBURNEY'S
ANOREXIA, FEVER, NAUSEA
(PERITONEAL)
↳ INVOLUNTARY GUARDING
↳ REBOUND TENDERNESS
DX : CT SCAN (ADULTS)
U/S   (KIDS)

TX : SURGERY
F/U : PO ABX NON-SEVERE
(CHILDREN) AMOX-CLAV

DIVERTICULAR DZ

FORMATION : TIME (40+), CONSTIPATION
PENETRATION THROUGH CIRCULAR M.
"NO" LONGITUDINAL M
FALSE DIVERTICULAR

SEROSA
BV
SUBMUCOSA   MUCOSA

DIVERTICULOSIS
ASX... FOUND ON SCREENING
COLONSCOPY FOR SOMETHING ELSE

DIVERTICULAR HEMORRHAGE
VISUALLY IMPRESSIVE (BRBPR)

SELF-LIMITING ... Ø△ HGB
PAINLESS   ... Ø△ HEMODYNAMICS

DIVERTICULITIS
PATH : "APPENDICITIS OF LEFT"
PT : ANOREXIA, FEVER, NAUSEA
LLQ ABD PAIN
(PERITONITIS)
DX : CT SCAN
COLONOSCOPY, 2-6 WKS LATER
TX : CIPRO + MTZ
SURGERY

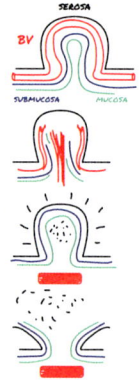

The Anatomy of the Abdominal Wall

EPIDERMIS	
DERMIS	

• HYPODERMIS
• SUBQ FAT
• CAMPER'S FASCIA

SUPERFICIAL ADIPOSE TISSUE   SAT
(CAMPER'S)
EVERYWHERE

══════════   ML (GARBAGE)

DEEP ADIPOSE TISSUE   DAT (SCARPA'S)
(ABD MUSCLES ONLY)

▬▬▬▬   FASCIA

MUSCLE

ABDO WALL MUSCLES

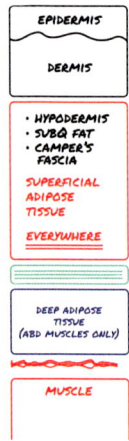

ANTERIOR
EXTERNAL OBLIQUE   EXTERNAL OBLIQUE
INTERNAL OBLIQUE = RECTUS ABDOMINIS   RECTUS = INT OBL
TRANSVERSALIS (TRANSVERSUS)   TRANSVERUS (TRANSVERSALIS)
TRANSVERSALIS FASCIA   TRANSVERSALIS FASCIA
POSTERIOR

ARCUATE LINE

ARCUATE LINE
INFERIOR V EPIGASTRIC A
RECTUS

RECTUS
EXTERNAL OBLIQUE
INTERNAL OBLIQUE
TRANSVERSALIS M. TRANSVERSALIS FASCIA

ARCUATE

RECTUS
EXT OBLIQUE
INT OBLIQUE
TRANSVERSALIS M. TRANSVERSALIS FASCIA

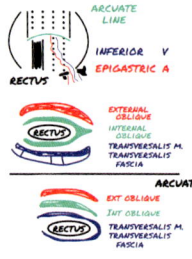

INGUINAL CANAL

INGUINAL LIG = APONEUROSIS OF MUSCLES
DEEP RING ABOVE ING. LIG.
AND LATERAL TO EPIGASTRIC

DEEP RING THE CANAL
SUPERFICIAL RING

SPERMATIC CORD

F.	TRANSVERSALIS FASCIA	INTERNAL CREMASTERIC FASCIA	F.
M.	INTERNAL OBLIQUE	CREMASTER	M.
M.	EXTERNAL	TRANSVERSUS	
"F."	EXTERNAL OBLIQUE	EXTERNAL CREMASTERIC FASCIA	F.
(BC)	PROCESSUS VAGINALIS	TUNICA VAGINALIS	(BC)

INGUINAL TRIANGLE

RECTUS
INFERIOR EPIGASTRIC A
DEEP RING
INGUINAL LIGAMENT
TRANSVERSALIS (TRANSVERSUS) FASCIA

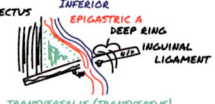

FEMORAL TRIANGLE △ ISH

NAVEL
LATERAL ──────→ MEDIAL

NERVE ARTERY VEIN
INGUINAL LIG.
SARTORIUS
ADDUCTOR
SHEATH   LYMPHATICS

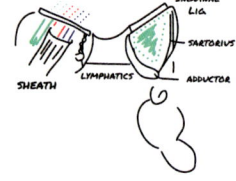

Gastrointestinal

Hernias and Small Bowel Obstruction

HERNIAS

INGUINAL
- ↳ **INDIRECT** = PROCESSUS VAGINALIS
  ♂, NEONATES, ABOVE INGUINAL LIG
  LATERAL TO EPIGASTRIC V.
  THROUGH THE DEEP INGUINAL RING
  SO IS WITHIN SPERMATIC CORD
- ↳ **DIRECT** = INGUINAL TRIANGLE
  ♂, ADULT, ABOVE INGUINAL LIG
  MEDIAL TO EPIGASTRIC L.

FEMORAL
- ↳ ♀ ADULT, BELOW INGUINAL LIG
  IN THE THIGH, IN FEMORAL TRIANGLE
  OUTSIDE THE FEMORAL SHEATH

VENTRAL
- ↳ POST-OP COMPLICATION
- ↳ FAILED HEALING OF MUSCLE LAYER

* UMBILICAL
- ↳ NEONATES, THROUGH UMBILICAL

HERNIA SEVERITY

① **REDUCIBLE**
SMALL DEFECT, LITTLE BOWEL
HERNIATES, EASILY REDUCED
ASX ELECTIVE REPAIR

② **INCARCERATED**
SMALL DEFECT, LOTS BOWEL
HERNIATED, NOT REDUCIBLE
IF SBO = URGENT, ELECTIVE

③ **STRANGULATED**
INCARCERATED + COMPROMISED
VASCULATURE = ISCHEMIA INFARCT
⊕POOP ⊕LACTATE = EMERGENCY

SBO IN GENERAL

PATH: MANY ETIOLOGIES...→
CHYME, GAS CANNOT PROGRESS
PT: EARLY = ABD PAIN COLICKY
(PERISTALSIS)
MID = CONSTANT ABD PAIN, N/V
DISTENDED + TYMPANITIC
BORBORYGMI (5 MINS)
LATE = OBSTIPATION, ABSENT
BOWEL SOUNDS
DX: UPRIGHT, KUB = AIR-FLUID LEVELS
CT SCAN = TRANSITION POINT
TX: NG TUBE INTERMITENT SUCTION
SURGERY

SELECTED CAUSES OF SBO

① **ADHESIONS**
MOST COMMON CAUSE OF SBO IF H/O SURGERY
OUTCOME OF HEALING (SCAR)

② **INCARCERATED HERNIA**
MOST COMMON CAUSE OF SBO IF NO SURGERY
⊕ HERNIA, NOT REDUCIBLE
∅ ECCHYMOSIS + ∅POOP

③ **INTUSSUSCEPTION**
TELESCOPING OF ONE BOWEL SEGMENT
INTO ANOTHER
KIDS: MECKEL'S   ADULTS: CANCER
VASCULATURE = ⊕ POOP, ⊕ LACTATE

④ **VOLVULUS**
TWISTING OF BOWEL AROUND ITSELF
(RECTUM, SIGMOID ADULTS... MALROTATION KIDS)
VASCULATURE = ⊕ POOP, ⊕ LACTATE

*⑤ **GALLSTONE ILEUS** (OBSTRUCTION)

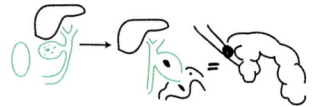

Physiology of Bile and Bilirubin

ANATOMY + FLOW

HEPATOCYTES MAKE BILE,
SECRETE INTO CANALICULI
CANALS OF HERING = STEM CELLS
CHOLANGIOCYTES = SIMPLE
COLUMNAR, LINE DUCTS

DUCTULES → DUCTS → ⓛ + ⓡ HEPATIC

AMPULLA ← COMMON BILE ⟨ CYSTIC
VATER   PANCREATIC GB

PHYSIOLOGY OF FLOW

HEPATO- ISOTONIC PRODUCTION OF
CYTES   BILE, RATE ≈ FIXED
   ↓BS 2/2 LOST BS, ↑RATE
GB   STORES BILE + EXTRACTS H_2O
CHOLAN-
GIOCYTE ↑CCK
   CONTRACTION = EJECTION INTO
DUODENUM

DUCT   FLUSHES ≈ AQUEOUS BICARBONATE
CHOLAN-   FLUID
GIOCYTE SECRETIN ↓
   MORE FLUID SECRETED

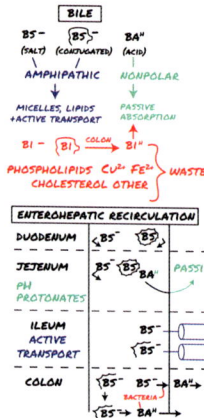

BILE

BS⁻   BS⁻   BA"
(SALT) (CONJUGATED) (ACID)
AMPHIPATHIC   NONPOLAR

MICELLES, LIPIDS   PASSIVE
+ACTIVE TRANSPORT ABSORPTION

BI⁻ — [BI] —COLON→ BI"

PHOSPHOLIPIDS $Cu^{2+} Fe^{2+}$ ⟩ WASTE
CHOLESTEROL OTHER

ENTEROHEPATIC RECIRCULATION

DUODENUM ⟨BS⁻ (BS⁻)
JEJENUM   BS⁻ (BS⁻) BA" PASSIVE
PH
PROTONATES
ILEUM   BS⁻
ACTIVE   BS⁻
TRANSPORT
COLON   ⟨BS⁻ BS⁻→ BA"⟩
   BACTERIA
   ⟨BS⁻→ BA"⟩

BILIRUBIN METABOLISM

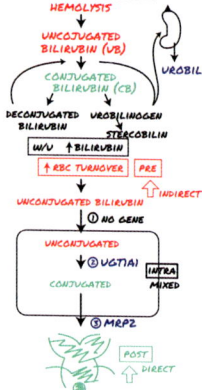

HEMOLYSIS

UNCOJUGATED
BILIRUBIN (UB)

CONJUGATED
BILIRUBIN (CB)   UROBILIN

DECONJUGATED UROBILINOGEN
BILIRUBIN   STERCOBILIN

W/U ↑BILIRUBIN

↑RBC TURNOVER PRE

UNCONJUGATED BILIRUBIN INDIRECT

① NO GENE
UNCONJUGATED
② UGT1A1   INTRA
CONJUGATED   MIXED
③ MRP2

POST DIRECT

NEONATAL JAUNDICE

PHYSIOLOGIC JAUNDICE
OF THE NEWBORN.
ASX, GONE BY 1ST CHECKUP

BREASTFEEDING JAUNDICE
↓MOTILITY, ↓FEEDING
FEED BABY MORE
BREAST - MILK JAUNDICED
ENZYME INHIBITS CONJUGATION?
FEED BABY FORMULA

CONGENITAL JAUNDICE

→ CN TYPE I = FATAL
ABSENCE OF UGT1A1
AR → DELETION
CN TYPE II = ASX ≈ SEVERE
AD → ↓ACTIVITY UGT1A1
   ↳ MANY FAM HX, LITTLE JAUNDICE
GILBERT'S
AR → ↓ ACTIVITY UGT1A1
ADULT JAUNDICE ≈ STRESS
DUBIN-JOHNSON = BLACK LIVER
AR → ↓ MRP2
LITTLE JAUNDICE ≈ STRESS
ROTOR'S = DJ ≈ BLACK
AR   LIVER

N O T E S

Gastrointestinal

Cholestasis

CHOLESTASIS - GENERAL

Bx: Bile Lakes, Plugs
Periportal Necrosis/Fibrosis

Labs: ↑ALP ↑Direct Bili

Sxs: ↑Bilirubin = Jaundice
↑Cholesterol = Xanthomas
↑Bile Salts = Pruritis

Extra-Hepatic	Intra-Hepatic
Stones (Acute)	PBC
Cancer (Painless)	"Metabolic"
PSC	Sepsis
	Estrogen
	Drugs

BILIARY CIRRHOSIS

Gall Stones Too Acute	Cancers Too Lethal

⬇

Autoimmune Cholangiopathies

"ESLD" ≃ Biliary Phenotype
(Cirrhosis) ↳ Large Green Liver
↳ Periportal Fibrosis
↳ Mallory-Denk Bodies
↳ Feathery, Balloon Degeneration

GALLSTONES

Cholesterol
Female   Green
Fat   Cholesterol
Forty
Fertile
Native American

Pigment
Hemolysis Black
           Bilirubin

CHOLELITHIASIS
Path: Gallstones NOT Stuck
Pt: Colicky, RUQ worse ⯠ Meals
U/S: Stones
Dx: N/A
Tx: Elective Removal

CHOLECYSTITIS
Stone Stuck
Cystic Duct
⊕ Murphy
Constant RUQ
+/- Mild Sepsis
Fluid, Stones, Thickened Wall
HIDA
Urgent Removal

CHOLEDOCHOLITHIASIS
Stone Stuck
CBD, Ø Inflame
Constant RUQ
↑LFTS Ø Sepsis
CBD Dilated
MRCP
Urgent Retrieval

GALLSTONE PANCREATITIS
Stone Stuck
Ampulla
"Pancreatitis"
+
↑LFTS
CBD Dilated
MRCP
Emergent Retrieval

ASCENDING CHOLANGITIS
Any + Infxn
Fever, Jaundice
RUQ ("Triad")
+
Hypo, AMS ("Pentad")
Dilated CBD
MRCP
Cx, Fluid, Abx
Emergent Retrieval

PRIMARY SCLEROSING CHOLANGITIS

Path: AIC Extra-Hepatic
Ducts. M. UC T_n/?
Ptn: ① ASX ↑ALP
     ② "Ascending Cholangitis"
Dx: MRCP = Beads on a String
    Liver-Bx Ductal-Bx
Tx: GI: Stent
    Transplant: Don't Stent
F/u: Onion-Skin Fibrosis
     On a Liver Bx
     Rarely Seen

PRIMARY BILIARY CIRRHOSIS

Path: AIC Intra-Hepatic
Ducts. W
Pt: ① Insidious Onset
    Fatigue + Pruritis, Jaundiced
    "To Yow" ⯠ Additional
    ② ASX ↑ALP + ↑D. Bili
Dx: AMA (ANA, ANCA)
    Liver Bx = Florid Ductal Lesion
    Lymphocytes Surrounding + Compressing Small Ducts + Macrophages
Tx: Ursodeoxycholic Acid
    Transplant
F/u: Fat ⟵ No ⟶ Hyper Bili
     Malabsorption Tx

BILIARY CANCERS

↳ Cholangiocarcinoma
Path: UC → PSC → Cholangio or Clonorchis Infxn
Pt: Painless Jaundice
    Progressive Insidious
Dx: MRCP
    Dx
Tx: Palliative
↳ GB Adenocarcinoma
"70 Yow" ⯠ Gallstones
Porcelin GB
Palpable, Enlarged, Painless

Metabolic Liver Disease

① HEPATOCELLULAR
⇑ AST ↑ALP
  ALT D. Bili

② CHOLESTASIS/OBSTRUCTION
⇑ AST ↑ALP
  ALT D. Bili

③ JAUNDICE HEMOLYSIS
↑ T. Bili

Muscle   "OSI"   "IG"
CK CPK   TP ALB   MM SPEP
          T. Bili D. Bili   HIV HIV
                          HEP^c HEP^c
2:1   AST ALT
ETOH   ALB ALP
or   GGT ↑
Cirrhosis Bone
100s
Acetaminophen
Aflatoxin
Acute Viral Hep
A Clot
Autoimmune
Hypotension

FHF
Insult + No ↻ → INR > 1.5 FHF
Dz → Hepatic Encephalopathy
Death → Transplant

CAUSE	PATHOGENESIS	GENE	SYSTEM	CIRRHOSIS...AND	Dx	Tx
VIRAL						
WILSON'S	Cu²⁺ Accumulation In All Tissues Deposition = Dysfxn Protein-Name	ATP7B	Cu²⁺ Metabolism EYES	Basal Ganglia Descemets = Kayser Fleischer Rings Membrane	1st: Serum Cu²⁺ Ceruloplasmin Urine Copper Bx: Mallory-Denk Pericentral ↑Cu²⁺↑	Penicillamine Transplant Cures
HEMOCHROMATOSIS	↓Hepcidin Iron Accumulation	HFE	Fe²⁺ Metabolism	"Bronze Diabetes" Dia CHF Pancreas Skin Liver	1st: Ferritin ↑1000s Serum Fe²⁺ Transferrin > 50% Gross: Chocolate Liver Bx: Periportal, Lipofuscin ↑Fe²⁺↑ Prussian Blue	Phlebotomy Transplant Curative
A1AT DEF.	PiMM = Normal PiMZ = Normal PiZZ = Disease	Protease-1 Misfolded	Alveoli :Elastase	COPD (Not Smoker)	Bx: PAS⊕ Macrophages	Transplant Curative
PSC **PBC** **ETOH**	Cholestasis Pericentral	Steatosis : ETOH Dehydrogenase → NADH → FA Synthesis → + ETOH Alcoholic : Necrosis → Acute Inflammation Hepatitis Steatofibrosis → Collagen			Bx: Pericentral Fibrosis Surrounding Steatosis Mallory-Denk Balloon Degeneration	
NAFLD **SOMETHING ELSE**	= ETOH ... ⯠ ETOH					

PT PTT
INR
TP ALB   ⟶ Chronic Dz
T. BILI D. BILI
AST ⨯ ALT ⟵ Acute Dz
   ALP

PRE
INTRA
POST

Gastrointestinal

HISTOLOGIC CIRRHOSIS

- FIBROSIS ₹ REGENERATING NODULES
- HEPATOCYTES ARE STEM CELLS
- CANALS OF HERING ARE ALSO STEM CELLS
  LIVER INTENSELY REGENERATIVE
- CAPILLARIZATION → PORTAL HTN
  - ↳ ITO CELLS => FIBROBLASTS
  - ↳ ENDOTHELIAL CELLS MIGRATE
    TO COLLAGEN
  - ↳ ↓ PERISINUSOIDAL SPACE,
    ↑ RESISTANCE

HYPERDYNAMIC CIRCULATION

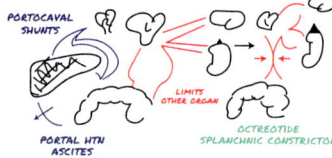

PORTOCAVAL SHUNTS

LIMITS OTHER ORGAN

PORTAL HTN
ASCITES

OCTREOTIDE
SPLANCHNIC CONSTRICTOR

HEPATIC ENCEPHALOPATHY

PATH: IMPAIRED UREA CYCLE
GUT BACTERIA=NH_3
NH_4^+ = TRAPPED

PT: AMS ASTERIXIS

DX: NH_3↑
CLINICAL

TX: LACTULOSE (2-3 BM/DAY)
RIFAXIMIN +/- ZINC

CLINICAL CIRRHOSIS

BILE
PRURITUS
JAUNDICE
XANTHOMA

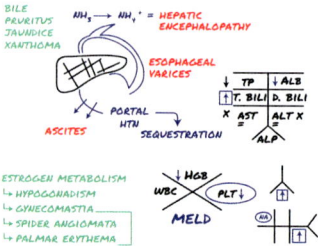

NH_3 → NH_4^+ = HEPATIC
ENCEPHALOPATHY

ESOPHAGEAL
VARICES

PORTAL
HTN
SEQUESTRATION

ASCITES

↓TP	↓ALB
↑T. BILI	D. BILI
X AST =	ALT X
	ALP

↓ ESTROGEN METABOLISM
↳ HYPOGONADISM
↳ GYNECOMASTIA
↳ SPIDER ANGIOMATA
↳ PALMAR ERYTHEMA

↓HGB
WBC X PLT↓

MELD

ASCITES

PATH: PORTAL HTN, J = K
PT: SHIFTING DULLNESS
FLUID WAVE
POCUS = BLACK
ABD DISTENSION

DX: U/S
DIAGNOSTIC PARA

TX: NACL <2 G/D + ALDO-ANTAG
H_2O <2 L/D   LOOP DIURETIC
THERAPEUTIC PARA (IV ALBUMIN)
~~TIPS~~

F/U: PPX FQ

ASCITES

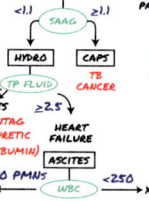

<1.1   ≥1.1
SAAG

HYDRO   CAPS

TP FLUID   TB
<2.5   CANCER
CIRRHOSIS
≥2.5

HEART
FAILURE

ASCITES

≥ 250 PMNS
SBP ←——— WBC ———→ X
<250

VARICES

PATH: PORTAL HTN
PT: ASX SCREENED EGD
OR
SEVERE BLEED

DX: EGD

TX: ACUTE:
OCTREOTIDE
BLAKEMORE TUBE
EGD, NO BB

CHRONIC:
NON-SELECTIVE BB
NADOLOL, PROPANOLOL

HCC

PATH: CIRRHOSIS (ANY)
HEP B

PT: ASX SCREENED
U/S + AFP

DX: TRIPLE PHASE CT

ARTERIAL

TX: MILAN
↳ RFA
↳ TRANSPLANT
↳ SORAFENIB

Gastrointestinal

Normal Kidney

Kidney Embryology

NOTES

Renal

Glomerular Filtration

20 MMHG — FILTRATION — REABSORPTION

MAP — 20 — ALL VESSELS — ART — RENIN → ANG 1 → ANG 2 → HTN — ADH — ALDO — ON

ANG 2 — JG CELLS — RENIN — NO — ANG 2 — RBF → ↑GFR — ↓TBF

GLOMERULAR — 50 — PERITUBULAR — FILTRATION — 50 — 20 — AFF — EFF — REABSORPTION

MYOGENIC RESPONSE — OFF — ON

TUBULOGLOMERULAR FEEDBACK
MD ↑GFR — JG CELLS — ADENOSINE CONSTRICTS ···↓GFR
MD ↑GFR — JG CELLS — RENIN — NITRIC OXIDE DILATES ···↑GFR

RBF / RPF — TBF — GFR — ↓TBF
RBF → ↑GFR ↑TBF — EFF — RBF → ↓GFR ↓TBF
↓RBF → ↓GFR ↓TBF — AFF — ↑RBF → ↑GFR ↑TBF
↑TBF — ↓TBF

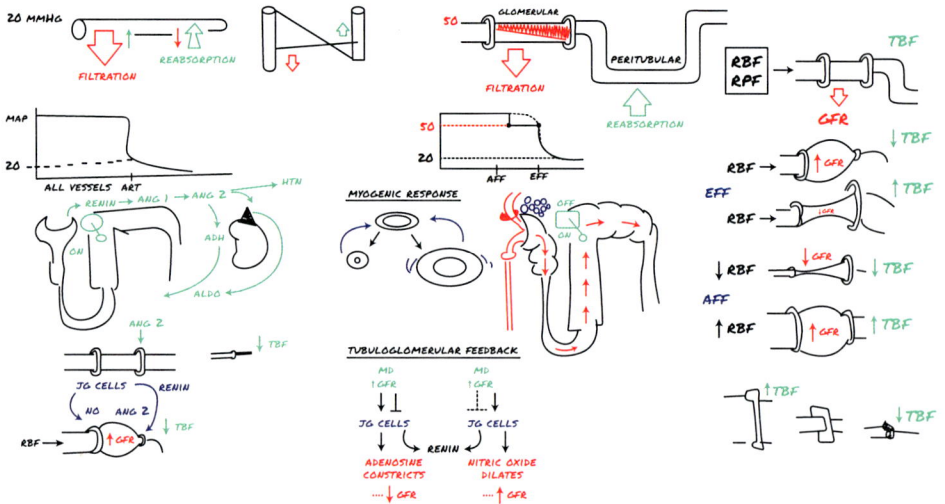

Regional Transport and Pharmacology

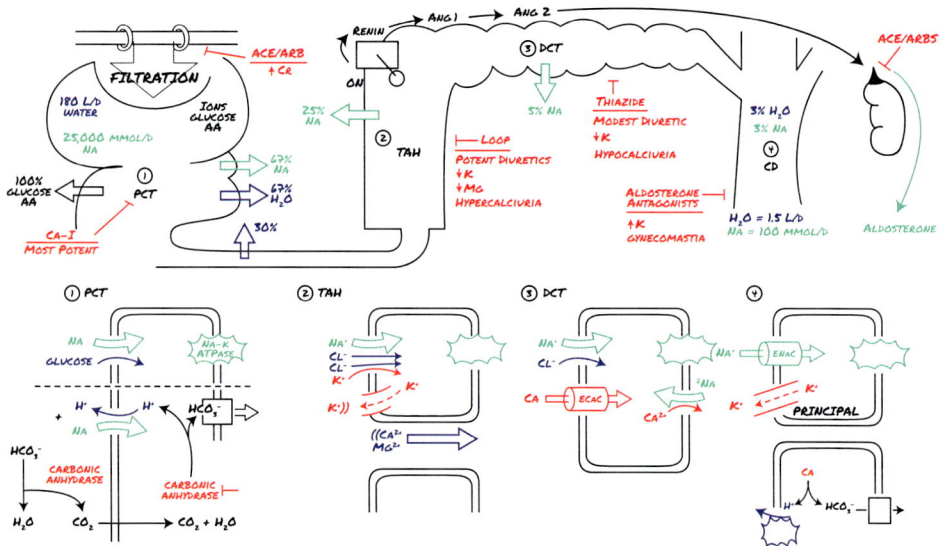

RENIN — ANG 1 — ANG 2 — ③ DCT — ACE/ARBS

FILTRATION — ACE/ARB ↑Cr — ON
180 L/D WATER — IONS GLUCOSE AA — 25% NA — ② TAH
25,000 MMOL/D NA — 5% NA — THIAZIDE MODEST DIURETIC ↓K HYPOCALCIURIA — 3% H₂O 3% NA — ④ CD
100% GLUCOSE AA — ① PCT — 67% NA — LOOP POTENT DIURETICS ↓K ↓Mg HYPERCALCIURIA — 67% H₂O — ALDOSTERONE ANTAGONISTS ↑K GYNECOMASTIA — H₂O=1.5 L/D NA=100 MMOL/D — ALDOSTERONE
CA-I MOST POTENT — 30%

① PCT: NA, GLUCOSE, NA-K ATPASE, H⁺, NA, HCO₃⁻, CARBONIC ANHYDRASE, H₂O, CO₂, CO₂+H₂O, CARBONIC ANHYDRASE, HCO₃⁻

② TAH: NA⁺, CL⁻, K⁺, K⁺), ((CA²⁺ Mg²⁺)

③ DCT: NA⁺, CL⁻, CA, ECAC, Ca²⁺, NA⁺, ²NA, K⁺

④: NA⁺ ENAC, K⁺ PRINCIPAL, CA, H⁺ HCO₃⁻

Renal

BALANCING CONCENTRATION GRADIENTS

WATER MOVES PASSIVELY   SOLUTE MOVES PASSIVELY

ESTABLISHING CONCENTRATION GRADIENT

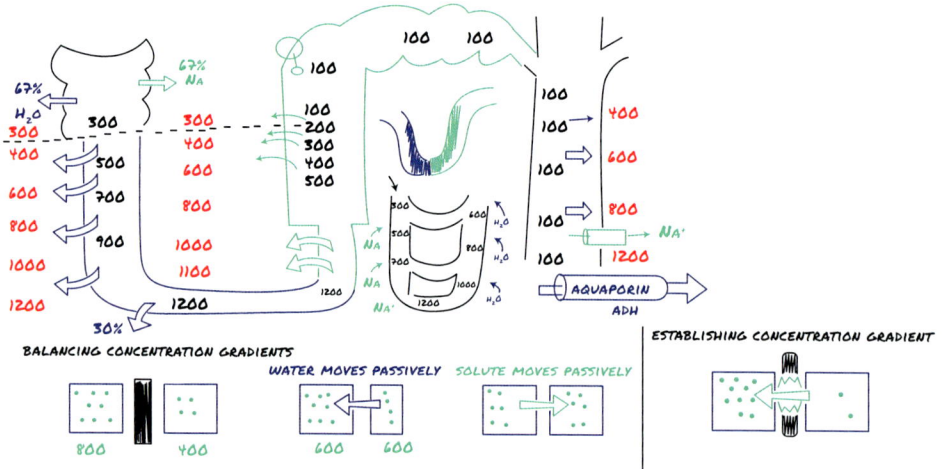

Kidney Stones

H⁺ HCO₃⁻ → ↑[CONSTITUENTS]

HYDRATION ALWAYS RIGHT

CALCIUM OXALATE | 67% STONES

OXALATE   Ca²⁺   ETHYLENE GLYCOL / VIT C

NEW MADE

OXALATE POOL

UNBOUND REABSORBED

FAT MALABSORPTION

UNBOUND ABSORBED

CA OXALATE NOT ABSORBED   CA OXALATE ELIMINATED

↑UOX
- BEANS, NUTS
- EXCESS VIT C
- ETHYLENE GLYCOL
- FAT MALABSORPTION

↑UCA
- LOOP DIURETICS
- HIGH-SALT DIET
+ THIAZIDE
+ CITRATE

CITRATE ↑UOX ↑UCA

ENVELOPE/DUMBELL

SMALL / ASX
MEDIUM / COLICKY FLANK PAIN / RADIATE TO GROIN / HEMATURIA
LARGE / +HYDRO / +↑CR

DIET + LIFESTYLE
<5 MM / FLUIDS / ANALGESIA
<10 MM / +MET
>10 MM / DISTAL: STENT / PROXIMAL: LITHOTRIPSY

X-RAY
CT SCAN (NONCONTRASTED) / STONE + HYDRO / V/A: ⊕ RBC
OR U/S / HYDRO / -STONE- → STRAIN CRYSTALS

STRUVITE
MAG AMMON ℗
UTI + UREASE ⊕
HUGE, ENVELOPE CALYCES / RADIO OPAQUE / COFFIN LID CRYSTALS
SURGERY
+ STAGHORN

URIC ACID
GOUT, LEUKEMIA
PURINE-RICH FOOD
SMALL / -LUCENT / RHOMBOID CRYSTALS
AVOID PURINE-RICH FOODS / PPX

CYSTINURIA
CHILDREN, STONE
COLA TRANSPORTER PCT
"SIXTINURIA" / HEXAGONAL CRYSTAL

CA P
OTHER CALCIUM
OTHER STAGHORN
HYPER PTH
WEDGE SHAPED

N O T E S

Cysts and Cancer

CORTEX + MEDULLA

ADPKD
PATH: AD, CHR 16
POLYCYSTIN = PKD1, PKD2
PT: CYSTS TOO SMALL = ASX
CYSTS GROW
  ↳ ESRD, YOUNG (50s)
  ↳ BERRY ANEURYSMS
  ↳ LIVER, PANCREAS
GROSS: MANY (B) CIRCULAR NONUNIFORM
HISTO: ROUND CYSTS Ž NORMAL GLOMERULI
PROG: ESRD, HD; TRANSPLANT

ACQUIRED POLYCYSTIC KIDNEY
PATH: ESRD/HD → CYSTS
  OBSTRUCTION TUBULAR FIBROSIS
GROSS: FEW, CIRCULAR CYSTS
HISTO: ——
PROG: PROGRESS TO RCC

CORTEX RCC

SIMPLE CYST
PATH: OBSTRUCTION OF DUCTS
PT: ASX, CORTICAL, SMALL

＊ RENAL CELL CARCINOMA
PATH: DELETION OF VHL, CHR 3
PT: ELDERLY SMOKER, MALES
10% {FLANK PAIN / FLANK MASS ← / HEMATURIA / HYPERTENSION}
GROSS: SINGLE YELLOW LESION
  UPPER POLE, LARGE
HISTO: CLEAR CELL
PROG: POOR, HEMATOGENOUSLY

VON HIPPEL–LINDAU
PATH: AD HYPERMETHYLATION VHL
PT: YOUNG (20s)
GROSS: MULTIPLE YELLOW
  THROUGHOUT KIDNEY
HISTO: SAA
ASSOC: HEMANGIOBLASTOMA — CEREBELLUM / RETINA

ONCOCYTOMA
RCC
Ø RCC

RENAL PAPILLARY ADENOMA
PATH: ≈ RCC

SINGLE YELLOW
  UPPER POLE, <3 CM
Bx Š NEPHRECTOMY

PARANEOPLASTIC
EPO = ↑HGB
RENIN = HTN
ACTH = CUSHING
  SYNDROME

MEDULLA

SPONGE KIDNEY
PATH: OBSTRUCTION COLLECTING DUCTS
GROSS: FEW CYSTS MEDULLA
ASSOC: PYELO + STONES

ANGIOMYOLIPOMA
TUBEROUS SCLEROSIS

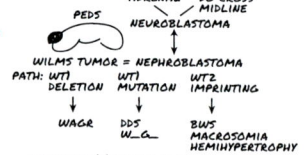

ADRENAL   DO CROSS
PEDS   MIDLINE
        NEUROBLASTOMA

WILMS TUMOR = NEPHROBLASTOMA
PATH: WT1   WT1   WT2
      DELETION   MUTATION   IMPRINTING

  WAGR   DDS   BWS
           W_G   MACROSOMIA
                     HEMIHYPERTROPHY

PT: YOUNG (5), FLANK MASS
  HYPERTENSION
GROSS: GREY TAN, LARGE
HISTO: ① STROMA
       ② ABORTIVE TUBULES
       ③ UNDIFFERENTIATED
         MESENCHYME
PROG: >90% 5 YR

Approach to Renal Failure

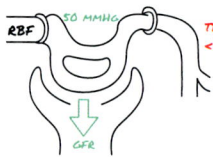

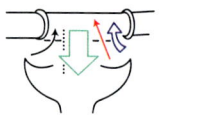

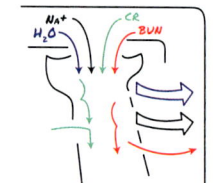

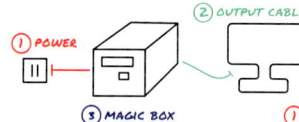

RBF   50 MMHG
TBF <20 MMHG   ① POWER
GFR
② OUTPUT CABLE
③ MAGIC BOX   ① PRE–RENAL   ③ MAGIC   ② POST–RENAL
                   PERFUSION   INTRARENAL   OBSTRUCTION

① PRE–RENAL = FILTRATION IMPAIRED, REABSORPTION INTACT
BUN
CR
BUN: CR > 20
PRE–RENAL
ON
RENIN → ANG 2 → ADH
            ALDOSTERONE
            ↓ UVOL
            ↑ UOSM > 300
Na² UNA < 10
    FENA < 1%

Na⁺
H₂O   CR   BUN

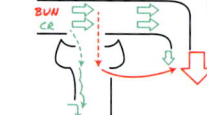

② POST–RENAL = FILTRATION IMPAIRED, REABSORPTION INTACT
HYDRO
U/S, CT SCAN   AKI
                  ARF
NOT LABS

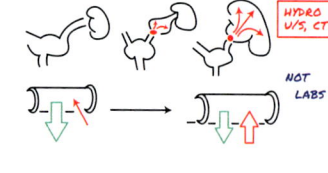

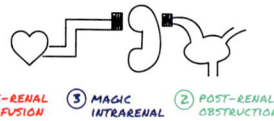

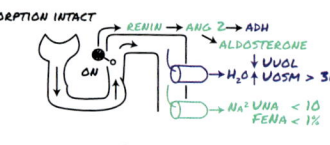

③ INTRARENAL = Bx
GLOMERULONEPHRITIS = RBC CASTS
            ACUTE   WAXY
            TUBULAR   BROWN
            NECROSIS   CASTS
            (ATN)

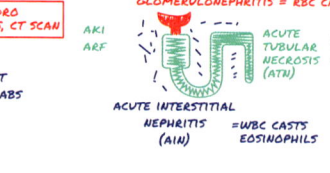

ACUTE INTERSTITIAL
NEPHRITIS   = WBC CASTS
(AIN)   EOSINOPHILS

Renal

Tubulointerstitial Diseases

ATN

TBF ✓ / RBF ✓ / GFR ✓

TBF ↓

Toxic = PCT
RHABDO (MYOGLOBIN), AMPHOTERICIN CONTRAST DYE

Ischemic = PCT, TAL, DCT

H_2O / IONS / BUN/CR / ↑CR

NORMAL	PRODROME	OLIGURIC	POLYURIC	NORMAL
	APOPTOSIS SLOUGHING EPITHELIUM	FILTRATION HYPERKALEMIA VOLUME OVERLOAD ↑BUN/↑CR < 10	REABSORPTION HYPOKALEMIA VOLUME DEPLETION ↑BUN/↑CR	

BUN/CR / IONS / H_2O → ... H_2O / IONS / BUN/CR

AIN   ABSCESS   **PYELONEPHRITIS**
FEVER, CVA TENDERNESS

PYELONEPHRITIS / UTI CYSTITIS

GRAM ⊖ ORGANISMS
URGENCY, FREQUENCY, DYSURIA
WBC = MACRO, PMN
WBC CASTS
URINE: GRAM ⊖ ORGANISMS
MICRO
U/A: LEUKOCYTE ESTERASE ⊕
NITRITES

ALLERGIC NEPHRITIS
EOSINOPHILS + FEVER + RASH
(URINE) EOSINOPHILIA (CBC)
DIURETICS → SULFUR → PCN CEPHALO TMP-SMX

NSAID = ↓PGE
ANG 2 / PGE ↓ANG 2
PAPILLARY NECROSIS
UROTHELIAL CARCINOMA PELVIS   FIBROSIS   HEMATURIA

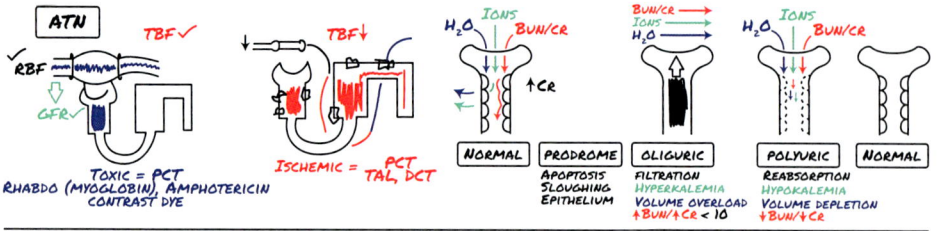

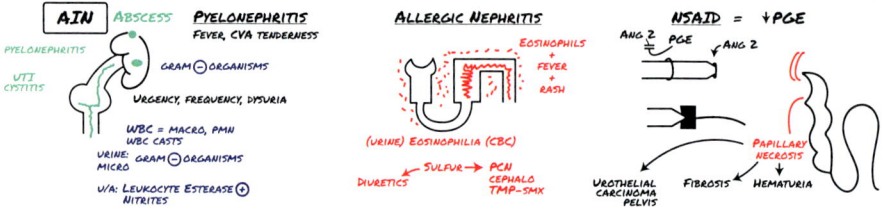

Introduction to Glomerulonephritis

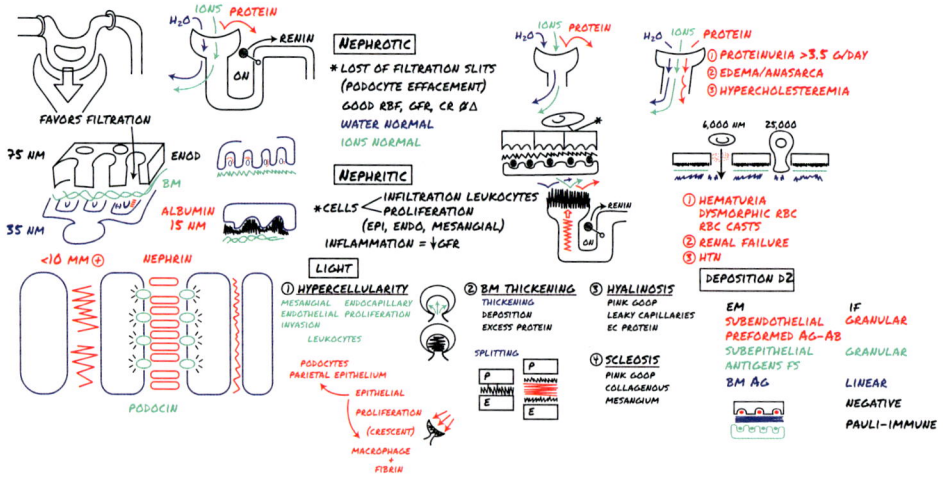

IONS / PROTEIN / H_2O → RENIN / ON
FAVORS FILTRATION
75 NM / ENOD / BM / ALBUMIN 15 NM
35 NM
<10 MM ⊕   NEPHRIN
PODOCIN

NEPHROTIC
* LOST OF FILTRATION SLITS
(PODOCYTE EFFACEMENT)
GOOD RBF, GFR, CR Ø Δ
WATER NORMAL
IONS NORMAL

NEPHRITIC
*CELLS ← INFILTRATION LEUKOCYTES
PROLIFERATION
(EPI, ENDO, MESANGIAL)
INFLAMMATION = ↓GFR

IONS / PROTEIN / H_2O RENIN / ON

H_2O IONS / PROTEIN
6,000 NM / 25,000

① PROTEINURIA >3.5 G/DAY
② EDEMA/ANASARCA
③ HYPERCHOLESTEREMIA

① HEMATURIA DYSMORPHIC RBC RBC CASTS
② RENAL FAILURE
③ HTN

LIGHT
① **HYPERCELLULARITY**
MESANGIAL   ENDOCAPILLARY
ENDOTHELIAL PROLIFERATION
INVASION
LEUKOCYTES
PODOCYTES
PARIETAL EPITHELIUM
EPITHELIAL
PROLIFERATION
(CRESCENT)
MACROPHAGE + FIBRIN

② **BM THICKENING**
THICKENING
DEPOSITION
EXCESS PROTEIN
SPLITTING
P | P / E | E

③ **HYALINOSIS**
PINK GOOP
LEAKY CAPILLARIES
EC PROTEIN

④ **SCLEOSIS**
PINK GOOP
COLLAGENOUS
MESANGIUM

DEPOSITION DZ

EM	IF
SUBENDOTHELIAL PREFORMED AG-AB	GRANULAR
SUBEPITHELIAL ANTIGENS FS	GRANULAR
BM AG	LINEAR
	NEGATIVE
	PAULI-IMMUNE

Renal

Nephrotic Syndrome

PODOCYTE EFFACEMENT SYNONYMOUS ℤ NEPHROSIS

H₂O / IONS / CR
PROTEIN → ALBUMIN
IG → AT3, c+5
PROTEIN FILTERED
NO INFLAMMATION

WATER / IONS / GFR — UNAFFECTED — ↑THROMBOSIS

① ALBUMINURIA >3.5G/DAY FROTHY
② EDEMA — ANASARCA
③ HYPERCHOLESTEREMIA MEMORIZE

PODOCYTE-SIDE GRANULAR
SUB-EPITHELIAL   ℤEMBRANOUS ③
PLANTED AG / PODOCYTE AG

EPI
ENDO

SUB-ENDOTHELIAL PREFORMED AG-AB GRANULAR   MPGN-I ①
MPGN-II ②   LINEAR RIBBON

NOT IMMUNE DEPOSITION — MCD
① NEPHROSIS OF KIDS
② RESPONSIVE TO STEROIDS
   LIMITED KNOWLEDGE

LM: NORMAL
EF: NEGATIVE
EM: EFFACEMENT

EM = EFFACEMENT — 1° FSGS
① MC NEPHROSIS IN U.S. HISPANICS
② RESPONSIVE TO STEROIDS
IDIOPATHIC, CONGENITAL, HIV HEROIN, SICKLE CELL

LM: SOME GLOMERULI WITH SOME SCLEROSIS
IF: NEGATIVE (IGM)
EM: EFFACEMENT

IF = NEGATIVE — 2° FSGS
SOME GLOMERULI DIE
COMPENSATORY HYPERTROPHY OF REMAINING
↑MAINTAIN GFR
↑PRESSURE CAPILLARY
INTRAGLOMERULAR HTN
MESANGIAL PROLIFERATION
PODOCYTE DENUDING

NOT IMMUNE DEPOSITION MEDIATED

MEMBRANOPROLIFERATIVE — MPGN TYPE I
PREFORMED AG-AB COMPLEXES
UNKNOWN AG
MESANGIAL PROLIFERATION INTO BM

LM: ENDOCAPILLARY, PROLIFERATION SPLITTING, BM THICKENING
EM: SUBENDO
IF: GRANULAR IGG + C3

DENSE DEPOSIT DZ — MPGN TYPE II
C3NEF = ANTIBODY
↑C3 CONVERTASE
MESANGIAL PRO INTO BM

LM: ENDOCAP PROLIFERATION SPLITTING BMT
EM: RIBBON-LIKE
IF: LINEAR C3

MEMBRANOUS NEPHROPATHY
"THREMBRANOUS" ℤEMBRANOUS
1° PLA₂ - RECEPTOR
2° PLANTED ANTIGENS HIV, HEP B, HEP C, SYPHILIS, GOLD, CAPTOPRIL, LUNG / COLON CA

LM: DIFFER CAPILLARY THICKENING
EM: SUBEPITHELIAL
IF: GRANULAR IGG + C3

Nephritic Syndrome

NEPHR**ITIS** = INFLAMMATION

ENTRY OF IMMUNE CELLS
25,000   6,000   15
WBC   RBC   PROTEIN
↓   ↓   X
GETTING INTO TISSUES HYPERCELLULARITY BX
HEMATURIA DYSMORPHIC RBC CASTS (5X5)

↓GFR
↑CR
OLIGURIC (5X5)
HTN

IONS / H₂O / PROTEIN
RENIN → ANG 2

APGN = **PSGN**

APGN:
ENDOCAPILLARY PROLIFERATION
INSTIGATED BY DEPOSITION OF PREFORMED AG-AB COMPLEXES
SUBENDOTHELIAL   ACUTE
SUBEPITHELIAL   INFLAMMATION
SELF-RESOLVE   MACRO, PMN
COMPLEMENT (C5A)

PSGN:
CHILD 6-8 YRS OLD
GETS A STREP INFXN THEN
2-4 WEEKS P̄ = NEPHRITIS
2/2 MPROTEIN
DON'T BX... SUPPORTIVE

LM: ENDOCAPILLARY PROLIFERATION
EM: SUBEPITHELIAL HUMPS
IF: GRANULAR IGM, IGG, COMP

IGA NEPHROPATHY
ENDOCAPILLARY PROLIFERATION
↑IGA DEPOSITION MESANGIUM
DURING - 2DAYS P̄ A MUCOSAL INFXN = NEPHRITIS
RECURRENT
LM: ENDO PROL
EM: MESANGIAL DEPOSITS
IF: IGA MESANGIUM

RPGN
EPITHELIAL PROLIFERATION
CRESCENTS → MACROPHAGES
   FIBRIN
DEPOSITION/IG
CELLS CRUSH GLOMERULAR TUFT, BREAKS BM
CM: CRESCENTS
EM: WRINKLED BM FRACTURED
IF: DEFINES DISEASE

RPGN - 1
LINEAR RPGN IS
GOOD PASTURE'S
ANTI-GBM ANTIBODIES
GLOMERULUS + ALVEOLAR
"
HEMATURIA + HEMOPTYSIS

ALPORT
NOT IMMUNE
X-LINKED RECESSIVE BOY
HEARING LOSS, POOR VISUAL ACUITY
NEPHRITIC SYNDROME

RPGN - 2
GRANULAR RPGN IS
LUPUS NEPHRITIS
PREFORMED AY-AB
COMPLEXES FORM
SUBENDOTHELIAL
PROGRESSION APGN

RPGN - 3
PAUCI-IMMUNE RPGN IS
A VASCULITIS
ALL ANCA ASSOCIATION
90% C-ANCA, ISOLATED
10% ANCA, RENAL + ELSE
WEGENER'S
   "C-ANCA PLUS"
   HEMOPTYSIS + ENT
   HEMATURIA
MICROSCOPIC POLYANGIITIS
   P-ANCA
CHURG-STRAUSS
   "P-ANCA PLUS"
   ASTHMA, EOSINOPHILIA

Renal

The Normal Bladder

OnlineMedEd

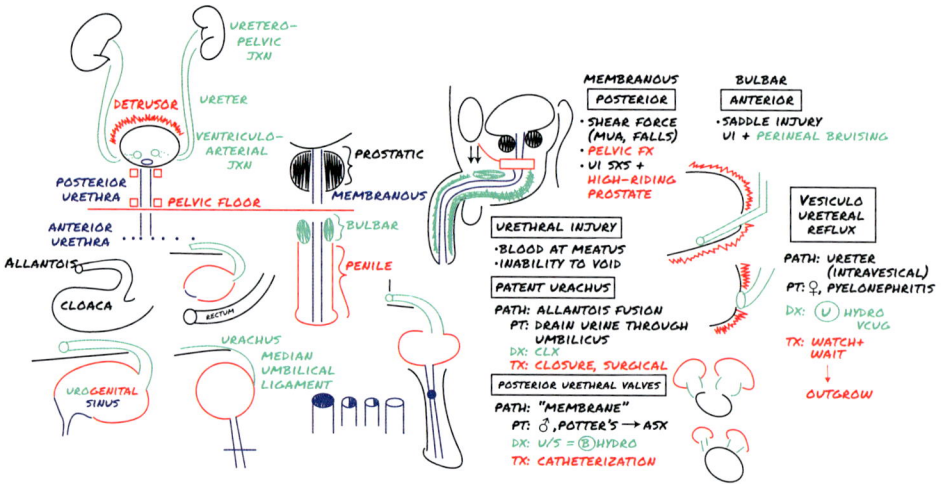

MEMBRANOUS
POSTERIOR
- SHEAR FORCE (MUA, FALLS)
- PELVIC FX
- UI SXS + HIGH-RIDING PROSTATE

BULBAR
ANTERIOR
- SADDLE INJURY
- UI + PERINEAL BRUISING

URETHRAL INJURY
- BLOOD AT MEATUS
- INABILITY TO VOID

PATENT URACHUS
PATH: ALLANTOIS FUSION
PT: DRAIN URINE THROUGH UMBILICUS
DX: CLX
TX: CLOSURE, SURGICAL

POSTERIOR URETHRAL VALVES
PATH: "MEMBRANE"
PT: ♂, POTTER'S → ASX
DX: U/S = Ⓑ HYDRO
TX: CATHETERIZATION

VESICULO URETERAL REFLUX
PATH: URETER (INTRAVESICAL)
PT: ♀, PYELONEPHRITIS
DX: Ⓤ HYDRO VCUG
TX: WATCH + WAIT
OUTGROW

Labels: URETERO-PELVIC JXN, DETRUSOR, URETER, VENTRICULO-ARTERIAL JXN, PROSTATIC, MEMBRANOUS, POSTERIOR URETHRA, PELVIC FLOOR, ANTERIOR URETHRA, BULBAR, PENILE, ALLANTOIS, CLOACA, RECTUM, URACHUS, MEDIAN UMBILICAL LIGAMENT, UROGENITAL SINUS

Micturition

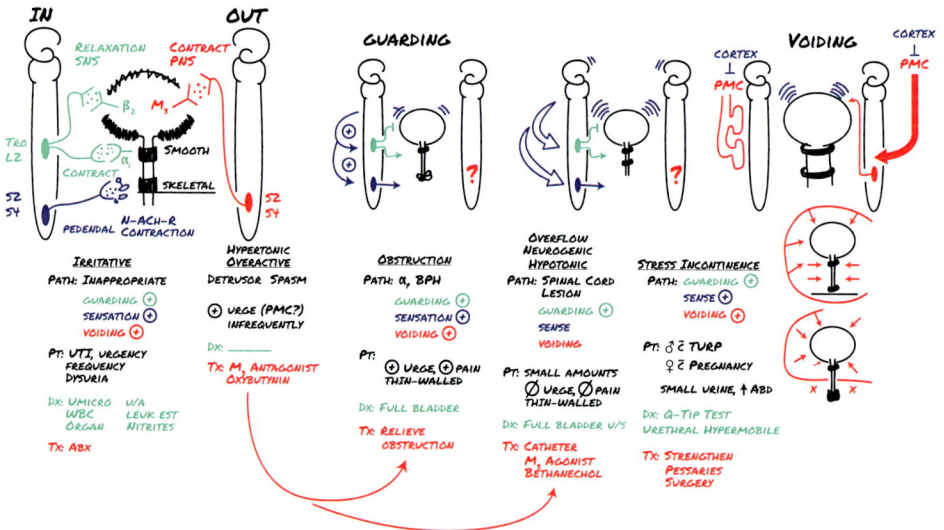

IN ... **OUT**
RELAXATION SNS, CONTRACT PNS, β₂, M₃, CONTRACT α, SMOOTH, SKELETAL, N-ACH-R PEDENDAL CONTRACTION, T₁₀ L₂, S₂ S₄

GUARDING   **VOIDING** CORTEX ⊥ PMC

IRRITATIVE
PATH: INAPPROPRIATE
GUARDING ⊕
SENSATION ⊕
VOIDING ⊕
PT: UTI, URGENCY FREQUENCY DYSURIA
DX: UMICRO WBC ORGAN W/A LEUK EST NITRITES
TX: ABX

HYPERTONIC OVERACTIVE
DETRUSOR SPASM
⊕ URGE (PMC?) INFREQUENTLY
DX: ___
TX: M₃ ANTAGONIST OXYBUTYNIN

OBSTRUCTION
PATH: α, BPH
GUARDING ⊕
SENSATION ⊕
VOIDING ⊖
PT: ⊕ URGE ⊕ PAIN THIN-WALLED
DX: FULL BLADDER
TX: RELIEVE OBSTRUCTION

OVERFLOW NEUROGENIC HYPOTONIC
PATH: SPINAL CORD LESION
GUARDING ⊕
SENSE ⊖
VOIDING ⊖
PT: SMALL AMOUNTS ∅ URGE, ∅ PAIN THIN-WALLED
DX: FULL BLADDER U/S
TX: CATHETER M AGONIST BETHANECHOL

STRESS INCONTINENCE
PATH: GUARDING ⊕
SENSE ⊕
VOIDING ⊕
PT: ♂ c̄ TURP ♀ c̄ PREGNANCY
SMALL URINE, ↑ABD
DX: Q-TIP TEST URETHRAL HYPERMOBILE
TX: STRENGTHEN PESSARIES SURGERY

94 © 2021 OnlineMedEd

N O T E S

Renal

95

Prostate

PROSTATE LOBES

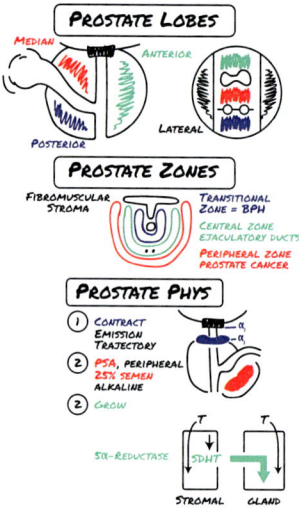

MEDIAN
ANTERIOR
LATERAL
POSTERIOR

PROSTATE ZONES

FIBROMUSCULAR STROMA

TRANSITIONAL ZONE = BPH
CENTRAL ZONE EJACULATORY DUCTS
PERIPHERAL ZONE PROSTATE CANCER

PROSTATE PHYS

1. CONTRACT EMISSION TRAJECTORY
2. PSA, PERIPHERAL 25% SEMEN ALKALINE
2. GROW

5α-REDUCTASE
5DHT
STROMAL   GLAND

BPH

PATH : BENIGN HYPERPLASIA
TRANSITIONAL ZONE

PT : OLD ♂ c̄ URINARY SXS
TRANSITIONAL ZONE
HESITANCY
INCOMPLETE VOIDING
DRIBBLING

DRE : SMALL, SINGULAR, RUBBERY
MOBILE NODULE

DX : CLX ... BX ... UNIFORM HYPERPLASIA

TX : (DILATE) α₁ – ANTAGONISTS
TAMSULOSIN   ORTHOSTATIC
HYPERTENSION

(SHRINK) 5α–REDUCTASE–I
FINASTERIDE   ↓LIBIDO
GYNECOMASTIA
TURP   TERATOGENIC

ACUTE PROSTATITIS

PT : "UTI"
DRE = TENDER, BOGGY, SWOLLEN
OLD ♂: GRAM ⊖ UTI
YOUNG ♂: GON/CHLA STI

PROSTATE CANCER

PATH : MALIGNANT ... INDOLENT GROWTH
PERIPHERAL ZONE

PT : SCREEN
OLD ♂ c̄ URINARY SXS
METASTASIS

DRE : LARGE, IRREGULAR, FIRM
FIXED, HARD NODULE

DX : PSA TRANSECTAL BX
NONUNIFORM HYPERPLASIA
SMALL NESTS OF "GLANDS"
GLEESON 2-10

TX : REJECTION
CASTRATION, CHEMICAL

F/U : PSA @ DIAGNOSIS
TRACK ... RESPONSE RELAPSE

ERECTILE DYSFUNCTION

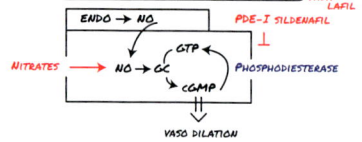

ENDO → NO
NITRATES → NO → GC → GTP → cGMP
PDE-I SILDENAFIL
PHOSPHODIESTERASE
TADA-LAFIL
VASO DILATION

Acid Base 1

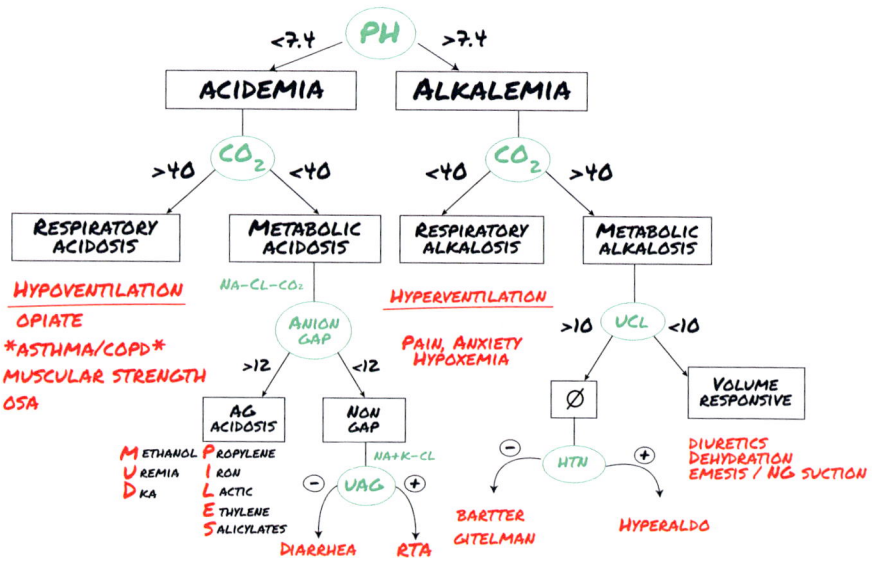

PH <7.4 >7.4

ACIDEMIA   ALKALEMIA

CO₂ >40 <40   CO₂ <40 >40

RESPIRATORY ACIDOSIS | METABOLIC ACIDOSIS | RESPIRATORY ALKALOSIS | METABOLIC ALKALOSIS

HYPOVENTILATION
OPIATE
ASTHMA/COPD
MUSCULAR STRENGTH
OSA

NA–CL–CO₂
ANION GAP
>12   <12

HYPERVENTILATION
PAIN, ANXIETY HYPOXEMIA

UCL >10 <10
Ø   VOLUME RESPONSIVE

AG ACIDOSIS | NON GAP

Methanol Propylene
Uremia   Iron
Dka   Lactic
         Ethylene
         Salicylates

NA+K-CL
UAG ⊖ ⊕
DIARRHEA   RTA

⊖ HTN ⊕
BARTTER   HYPERALDO
GITELMAN

DIURETICS
DEHYDRATION
EMESIS / NG SUCTION

Renal

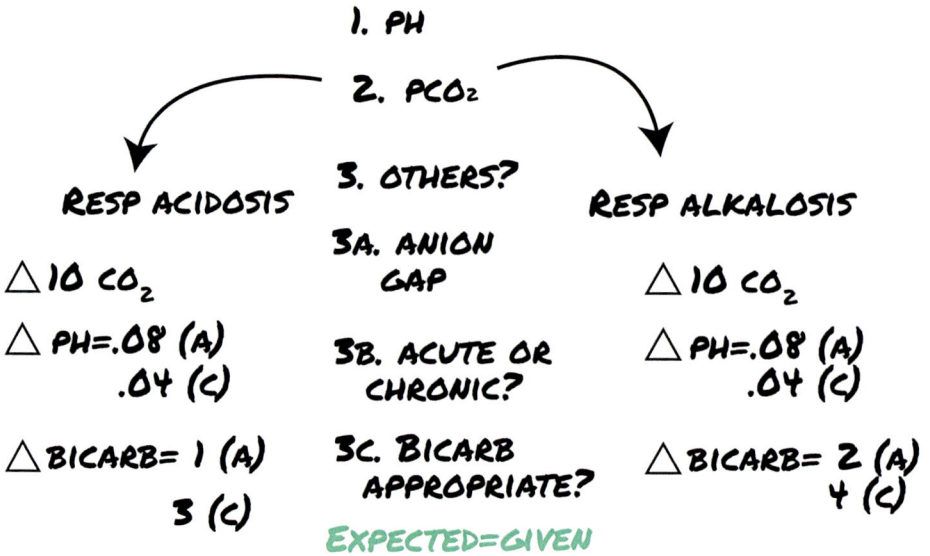

1. PH

2. PCO_2

3. OTHERS?

3A. ANION GAP

3B. ACUTE OR CHRONIC?

3C. BICARB APPROPRIATE?

EXPECTED=GIVEN

RESP ACIDOSIS

△ 10 CO_2

△ PH=.08 (A)
      .04 (C)

△ BICARB= 1 (A)
          3 (C)

RESP ALKALOSIS

△ 10 CO_2

△ PH=.08 (A)
      .04 (C)

△ BICARB= 2 (A)
          4 (C)

NOTES

Introduction to Hematology-Oncology

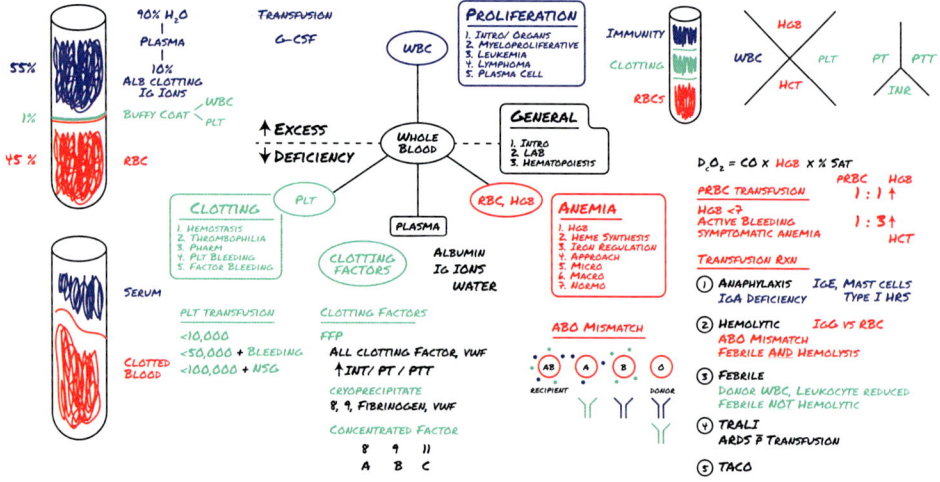

OnlineMedEd

90% H₂O
PLASMA
10%
ALB CLOTTING
IG IONS
BUFFY COAT — WBC
PLT

55%
1%
45%

RBC

SERUM

CLOTTED BLOOD

TRANSFUSION
G-CSF

↑ EXCESS
↓ DEFICIENCY

WBC

WHOLE BLOOD

PLT

PLASMA

CLOTTING
1. HEMOSTASIS
2. THROMBOPHILIA
3. PHARM
4. PLT BLEEDING
5. FACTOR BLEEDING

CLOTTING FACTORS

RBC, HGB

ALBUMIN
IG IONS
WATER

PROLIFERATION
1. INTRO/ ORGANS
2. MYELOPROLIFERATIVE
3. LEUKEMIA
4. LYMPHOMA
5. PLASMA CELL

IMMUNITY

CLOTTING

RBCs

GENERAL
1. INTRO
2. LAB
3. HEMATOPOIESIS

ANEMIA
1. HGB
2. HEME SYNTHESIS
3. IRON REGULATION
4. APPROACH
5. MICRO
6. MACRO
7. NORMO

HGB
WBC   PLT   PT   PTT
HCT   INR

$D_aO_2 = CO \times HGB \times \% SAT$

PRBC TRANSFUSION   PRBC   HGB
HGB <7   1 : 1 ↑
ACTIVE BLEEDING   1 : 3 ↑
SYMPTOMATIC ANEMIA   HCT

TRANSFUSION RXN
① ANAPHYLAXIS   IGE, MAST CELLS
   IGA DEFICIENCY   TYPE I HRS
② HEMOLYTIC   IGG VS RBC
   ABO MISMATCH
   FEBRILE AND HEMOLYSIS
③ FEBRILE
   DONOR WBC, LEUKOCYTE REDUCED
   FEBRILE NOT HEMOLYTIC
④ TRALI
   ARDS p̄ TRANSFUSION
⑤ TACO

PLT TRANSFUSION
<10,000
<50,000 + BLEEDING
<100,000 + NSG

CLOTTING FACTORS
FFP
ALL CLOTTING FACTOR, VWF
↑ INT/ PT / PTT
CRYOPRECIPITATE
8, 9, FIBRINOGEN, VWF
CONCENTRATED FACTOR
8   9   11
A   B   C

ABO MISMATCH
AB   A   B   O
RECIPIENT   DONOR

Laboratory Interpretation

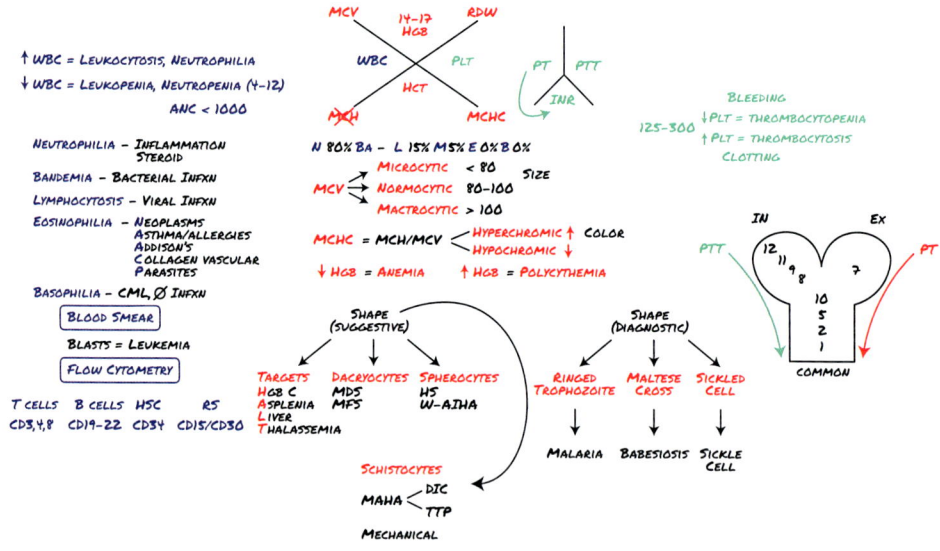

↑ WBC = LEUKOCYTOSIS, NEUTROPHILIA
↓ WBC = LEUKOPENIA, NEUTROPENIA (4-12)
         ANC < 1000

NEUTROPHILIA – INFLAMMATION
              STEROID
BANDEMIA – BACTERIAL INFXN
LYMPHOCYTOSIS – VIRAL INFXN
EOSINOPHILIA – NEOPLASMS
              ASTHMA/ALLERGIES
              ADDISON'S
              COLLAGEN VASCULAR
              PARASITES
BASOPHILIA – CML, Ø INFXN

[BLOOD SMEAR]
BLASTS = LEUKEMIA

[FLOW CYTOMETRY]

T CELLS   B CELLS   HSC   RS
CD3,4,8   CD19-22   CD34   CD15/CD30

MCV   14-17   RDW
       HGB
WBC   PLT
       HCT
MCH   MCHC

PT   PTT
     INR

N 80% BA – L 15% MS% E 0% B 0%

              Microcytic   < 80
MCV →   Normocytic   80-100   SIZE
              Macrocytic   > 100

MCHC = MCH/MCV ⟨ HYPERCHROMIC ↑ COLOR
                 HYPOCHROMIC ↓
↓ HGB = ANEMIA   ↑ HGB = POLYCYTHEMIA

BLEEDING
125-300   ↓ PLT = THROMBOCYTOPENIA
          ↑ PLT = THROMBOCYTOSIS
          CLOTTING

IN   EX
12   PT
11   7
9 8
10
5
2
1
COMMON

SHAPE (SUGGESTIVE)

TARGETS   DACRYOCYTES   SPHEROCYTES
HGB C   MDS   HS
ASPLENIA   MFS   W-AIHA
LIVER
THALASSEMIA

SHAPE (DIAGNOSTIC)

RINGED   MALTESE   SICKLED
TROPHOZOITE   CROSS   CELL
    ↓   ↓   ↓
MALARIA   BABESIOSIS SICKLE
                         CELL

SCHISTOCYTES
         ⟨ DIC
MAHA   TTP
MECHANICAL

Hematology Oncology

Hemoglobin

HEMOGLOBIN

β β + α α

GLOBIN TETRAMER ⇓ HEME

HEMOGLOBIN
$\alpha_2\beta_2$ = HBA$_1$ (98%) — ADULT
$\alpha_2\delta_2$ = HBA$_2$ (2%)
$\alpha_2\gamma_2$ = HBF → FETAL

%SAT

LUNGS RELAXED UPTAKE

50%

TISSUES

UNLOADING   15 (ACTIVE)   25 40 (REST) 60 80 100 P_AO_2

TAUT

AFFINITY   1   2   16   48   52

POSITIVE COOPERATIVITY

V_{MAX} ↑AFFINITY UPTAKE   ↑AFFINITY UNLOAD

HBF 2,3-BPG

2,3-BPG ↓PH CO_2 ↑TEMP

RELAXED K_M 1/AFFINITY

RELAXED RESPIRATORY   TAUT TISSUES

YOLK SAC LIVER SPLEEN BONE MARROW
α
β
γ
λ
ε

6 WEEKS   BIRTH   6 MONTHS

GLOBIN
α - GLOBIN CHR 16 4 COPIES
β - GLOBIN CHR 11 2 COPIES

HEME

SUCCINYL COA + GLYCINE   MITOCHONDRIA   HEME

B_6 D-ALA SYNTHETASE   HEME GLUCOSE   FERROCHELATASE

D-ALA   PROTO-PORPHYRIN-OGEN Fe^{2+}

CYTOPLASM SOME STUFF HAPPENS

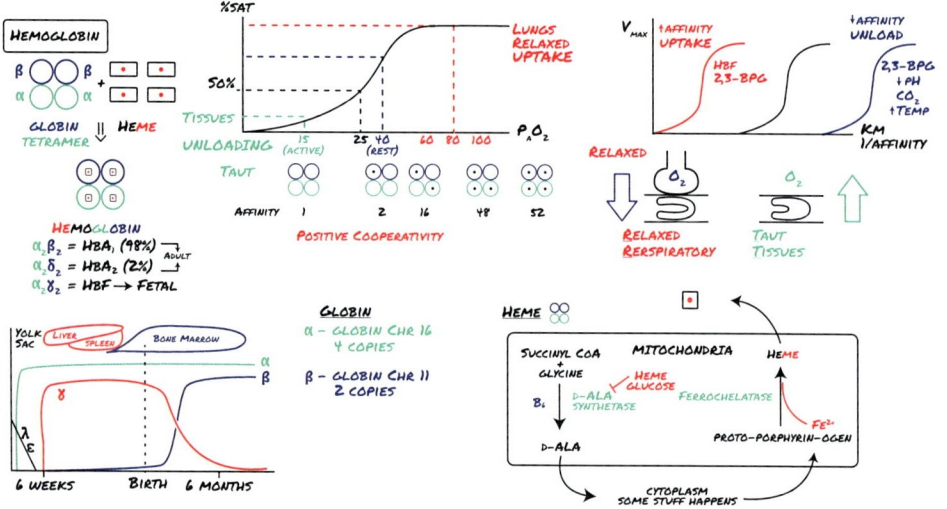

Disorders of Heme Synthesis

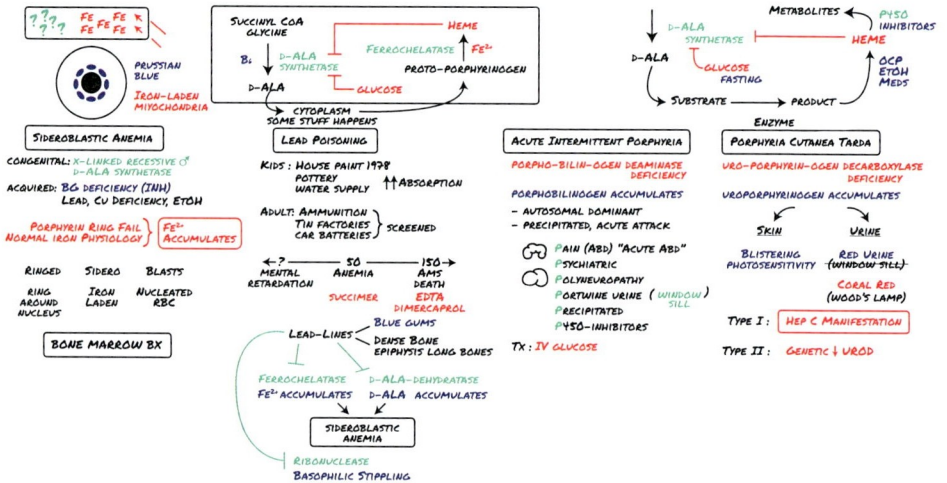

?? ?? FE FE FE
?? ?? FE FE FE

PRUSSIAN BLUE
IRON-LADEN MIYOCHONDRIA

SIDEROBLASTIC ANEMIA

CONGENITAL: X-LINKED RECESSIVE ♂ D-ALA SYNTHETASE
ACQUIRED: B6 DEFICIENCY (INH) LEAD, CU DEFICIENCY, ETOH

PORPHYRIN RING FAIL Fe^{2+}
NORMAL IRON PHYSIOLOGY   ACCUMULATES

RINGED   SIDERO   BLASTS
RING AROUND NUCLEUS   IRON LADEN   NUCLEATED RBC

BONE MARROW BX

SUCCINYL COA GLYCINE   HEME
B_6 D-ALA SYNTHETASE   FERROCHELATASE Fe^{2+}
D-ALA   PROTO-PORPHYRINOGEN
GLUCOSE
CYTOPLASM SOME STUFF HAPPENS

LEAD POISONING

KIDS: HOUSE PAINT 1978
POTTERY
WATER SUPPLY   ↑↑ABSORPTION

ADULT: AMMUNITION
TIN FACTORIES   SCREENED
CAR BATTERIES

←?——— 50 ———— 150→
MENTAL   ANEMIA   AMS
RETARDATION   DEATH
SUCCIMER   EDTA DIMERCAPROL
BLUE GUMS
LEAD-LINES DENSE BONE
EPIPHYSIS LONG BONES

FERROCHELATASE   D-ALA-DEHYDRATASE
Fe^{2+} ACCUMULATES   D-ALA ACCUMULATES

SIDEROBLASTIC ANEMIA

RIBONUCLEASE
BASOPHILIC STIPPLING

↓ D-ALA SYNTHETASE
D-ALA   GLUCOSE FASTING
SUBSTRATE ——— PRODUCT
ENZYME

METABOLITES ← P450 INHIBITORS
HEME

OCP ETOH MEDS

ACUTE INTERMITTENT PORPHYRIA

PORPHO-BILIN-OGEN DEAMINASE DEFICIENCY

PORPHOBILINOGEN ACCUMULATES
- AUTOSOMAL DOMINANT
- PRECIPITATED, ACUTE ATTACK

PAIN (ABD) "ACUTE ABD"
PSYCHIATRIC
POLYNEUROPATHY
PORTWINE URINE (WINDOW SILL)
PRECIPITATED
P450-INHIBITORS

TX: IV GLUCOSE

PORPHYRIA CUTANEA TARDA

URO-PORPHYRIN-OGEN DECARBOXYLASE DEFICIENCY

UROPORPHYRINOGEN ACCUMULATES

SKIN   URINE
BLISTERING   RED URINE
PHOTOSENSITIVITY   (WINDOW SILL)
CORAL RED
(WOOD'S LAMP)

TYPE I: HEP C MANIFESTATION
TYPE II: GENETIC ↓ UROD

Hematology Oncology

Iron Regulation

Fe^{2+} Fe^{3+}

EPO
Fe
IL-6
HYPOXIA

DMT1 MOBILFERRIN

HEPCIDIN

DUODENAL ENTEROCYTE

FERROPORTIN   FERROPORTIN

HEMOSIDERIN

UNCONJUGATED BILI

TRANSFERRIN

TIBC
HEPCIDIN
FERRITIN

EPO
C
HGB
FE

FERRITIN

FERROPORTIN   HEPCIDIN   FERRITIN
IRON
TRANSFERRIN   (TIBC)
% SATURATION

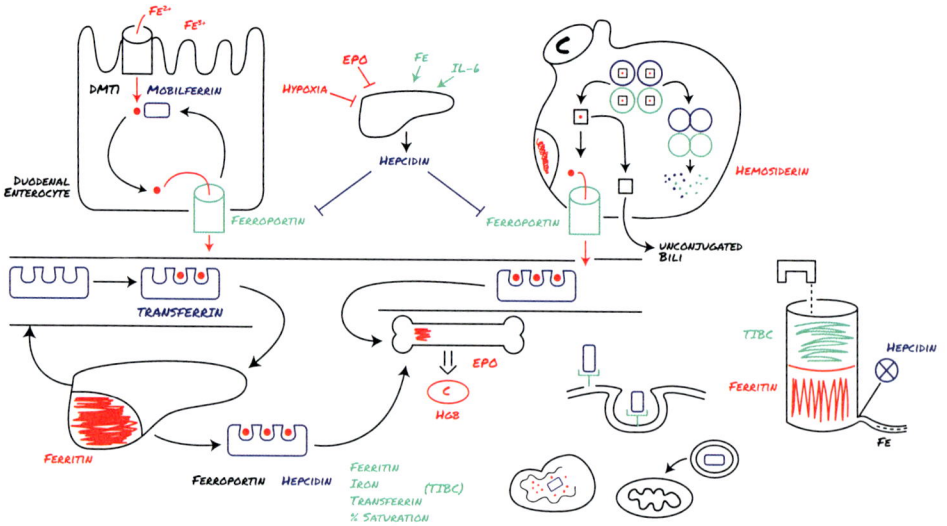

Approach to Anemia

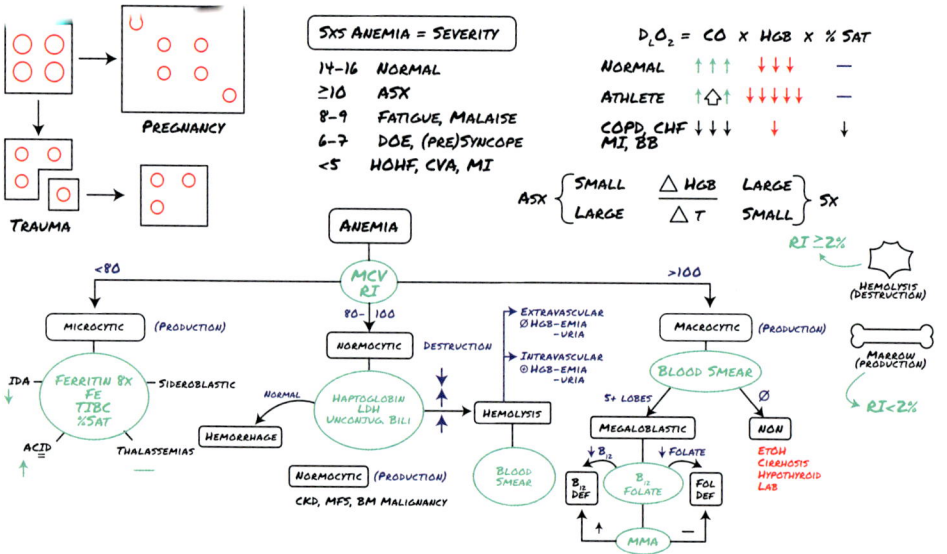

SXS ANEMIA = SEVERITY

14-16   NORMAL
≥10   ASX
8-9   FATIGUE, MALAISE
6-7   DOE, (PRE)SYNCOPE
<5   HOHF, CVA, MI

$D_2O_2 = CO \times HGB \times \% SAT$

NORMAL	↑↑↑	↓↓↓	—
ATHLETE	↑△↑	↓↓↓↓↓	—
COPD, CHF MI, BB	↓↓↓	↓	↓

ASX { SMALL / LARGE } △HGB / △T { LARGE / SMALL } SX

RI ≥2%

HEMOLYSIS (DESTRUCTION)

PREGNANCY

TRAUMA

ANEMIA

MCV
RI

<80   80-100   >100

MICROCYTIC (PRODUCTION)   NORMOCYTIC   DESTRUCTION   MACROCYTIC (PRODUCTION)

IDA — FERRITIN ↑x
↓   FE
TIBC
%SAT — SIDEROBLASTIC

NORMAL

ACID
=   HAPTOGLOBIN
LDH
THALASSEMIAS   UNCONJ. BILI

HEMORRHAGE

EXTRAVASCULAR
∅ HGB-EMIA
-URIA

INTRAVASCULAR
⊕ HGB-EMIA
-URIA

HEMOLYSIS

BLOOD SMEAR

MARROW (PRODUCTION)

RI < 2%

BLOOD SMEAR   5+ LOBES   ∅

MEGALOBLASTIC   NON

↓ B12   ↓ FOLATE   ETOH
CIRRHOSIS
HYPOTHYROID
LAB

NORMOCYTIC (PRODUCTION)   B12   B12   FOL
DEF   FOLATE DEF
CKD, MFS, BM MALIGNANCY

MMA

Hematology Oncology

Microcytic Anemia

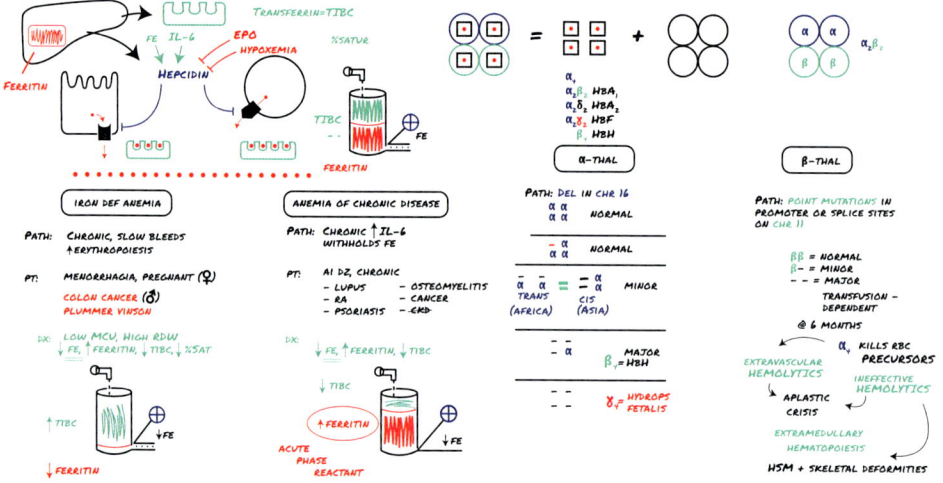

TRANSFERRIN = TIBC

FE   IL-6   EPO
            HYPOXEMIA

%SATUR

FERRITIN

HEPCIDIN

TIBC
- -   ⊕ FE

FERRITIN

- - - - - - - - - - - -

IRON DEF ANEMIA

PATH: CHRONIC, SLOW BLEEDS
↑ ERYTHROPOIESIS

PT: MENORRHAGIA, PREGNANT (♀)
COLON CANCER (♂)
PLUMMER VINSON

DX: LOW MCV, HIGH RDW
↓ FE, ↑ FERRITIN, ↓ TIBC, ↓ %SAT

↑ TIBC   ⊕
              ↓ FE

↓ FERRITIN

ANEMIA OF CHRONIC DISEASE

PATH: CHRONIC ↑ IL-6
WITHHOLDS FE

PT: AI DZ, CHRONIC
- LUPUS   - OSTEOMYELITIS
- RA   - CANCER
- PSORIASIS   - CKD

DX: ↓ FE, ↑ FERRITIN, ↓ TIBC
↓ TIBC

↑ FERRITIN   ⊕
              ↓ FE

ACUTE
PHASE
REACTANT

α_1
$\alpha_2\delta_1$ HBA$_1$
$\alpha_2\delta_2$ HBA$_2$
$\alpha_2\delta_2$ HBF
β_4 HBH

α-THAL

PATH: DEL IN CHR 16

$\frac{\alpha\ \alpha}{\alpha\ \alpha}$ NORMAL

$\frac{-\ \alpha}{\alpha\ \alpha}$ NORMAL

$\frac{\alpha\ \alpha}{-\ -}$ = $\frac{-\ \alpha}{-\ \alpha}$ MINOR
TRANS   CIS
(AFRICA)   (ASIA)

$\frac{-\ -}{-\ \alpha}$ MAJOR
β_4 = H8H

$\frac{-\ -}{-\ -}$ γ_4 = HYDROPS FETALIS

$\alpha\ \alpha$ $\alpha_2\beta_1$
$\beta\ \beta$

β-THAL

PATH: POINT MUTATIONS IN PROMOTER OR SPLICE SITES ON CHR 11

$\beta\beta$ = NORMAL
$\beta-$ = MINOR
$- -$ = MAJOR
TRANSFUSION - DEPENDENT
@ 6 MONTHS

α_4 KILLS RBC PRECURSORS

EXTRAVASCULAR   INEFFECTIVE
HEMOLYTICS   HEMOLYTICS

APLASTIC
CRISIS

EXTRAMEDULLARY
HEMATOPOIESIS

HSM + SKELETAL DEFORMITIES

Macrocytic Anemia

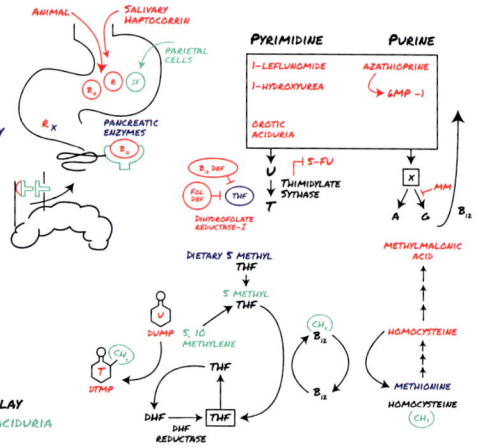

3-6 WEEKS

FOLATE DEF

CAUSE : LEAFY GREENS
(TEA + TOAST, ETOH)
JEJUNUM LESION (SPRUE)

↑ ERYTHROPOIESIS
- PREGNANCY
- CHRONIC HEMOLYTIC ANEMIA

PT: MEGALOBLASTIC ANEMIA

DX: ↓ FOLATE, ØDMMA

TX : FOLATE

10 YRS

B$_{12}$ DEF

CAUSES : VEGANISM, SJOGRENS
☆ PERNICIOUS ANEMIA
(GASTRIC SURGERY)
PANCREATIC INSUFFICIENCY
☆ TERMINAL ILEUM
TAPEWORM

PT: MEGALOBLASTIC ANEMIA
+ NEUROLOGIC SXS

DX: ↓ B$_{12}$, ↑ MMA

TX : B$_{12}$ (IM)
B$_{12}$ (PO)

RBC "MACROCYTIC"	PMN "MEGALOBLASTIC"
↓ NUCLEIC ACIDS	↓ NUCLEIC ACIDS
FEWER DIVISIONS	DELAYED DEVELOPMENT
↑ SIZE, ↓ RBC	NUCLEUS
Ø △ TIME TO DIFF	5+ LOBES
	Ø △ CYTOPLASM

OROTIC ACIDURIA

MEGALOBLASTIC
ANEMIA

AND

NEONATE, FTT
DEVELOPMENTAL DELAY

DX : URINE = OROTIC ACIDURIA
TX : UMP

ANIMAL   SALIVARY
              HAPTOCORRIN

PARIETAL
CELLS

R x

PANCREATIC
ENZYMES

PYRIMIDINE	PURINE
1-LEFLUNOMIDE	AZATHIOPRINE
1-HYDROXYUREA	↓ 6MP ⊣
OROTIC ACIDURIA	

B$_{12}$ DEF
FOL DEF THF

⊣ 5-FU
THIMIDYLATE
SYTHASE

DIHYDROFOLATE
REDUCTASE-1

X   MMA

A   G   B$_{12}$

METHYLMALONIC
ACID

DIETARY 5 METHYL
THF

5 METHYL
THF

DUMP 5, 10
METHYLENE

B$_{12}$

HOMOCYSTEINE

THF

B$_{12}$

METHIONINE
HOMOCYSTEINE (CH$_3$)

CH$_2$
DUMP
DUTMP

DHF   THF
DHF
REDUCTASE

Normocytic Anemia

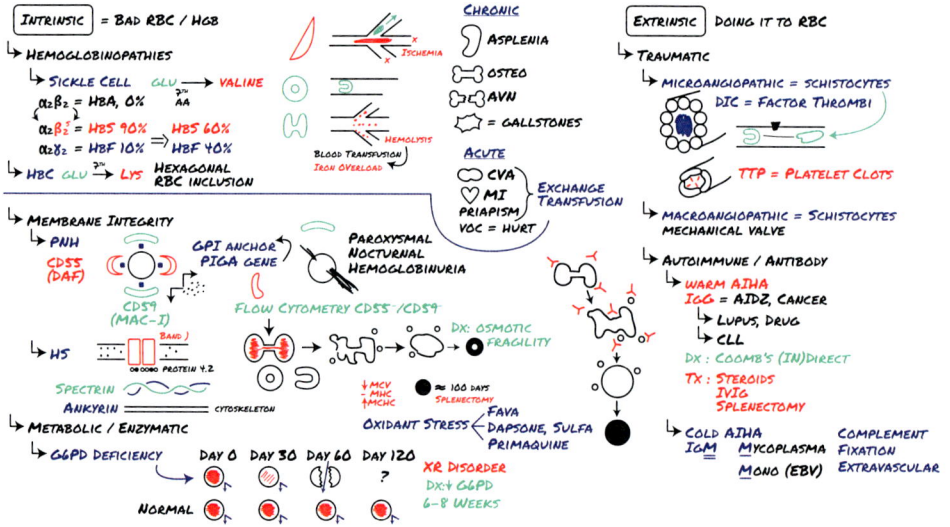

Hemostasis

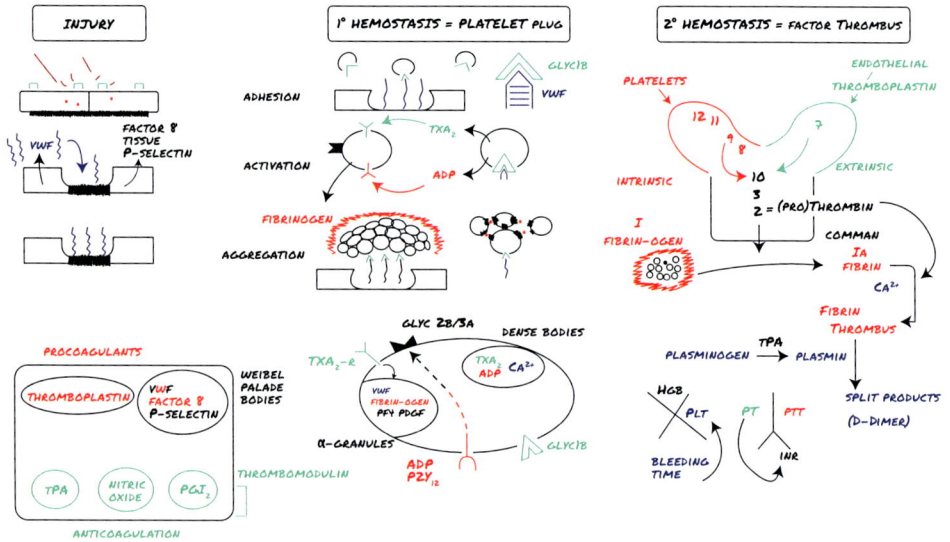

NOTES

Hematology Oncology

PRO — UNACTIVATED

PRO — ACTIVATED

INACTIVATED

THROMBOMODULIN

C

INTRINSIC
PLATELET PLUG

EXTRINSIC
THROMBOPLASTIN

12
11
9
9 7 7
10
8
8
5
C
5
5

PROTHROMBIN G20210A
PROTHROMBIN
2
THROMBIN
2
5
FACTOR V LEIDEN

HEPARIN
ANTITHROMBIN

FIBRINOGEN → FIBRIN → THROMBUS → SPLIT PRODUCTS
TPA

PROTEIN C, PROTEIN S ANTICOAGS SHORTER $T_{1/2}$

VITAMIN K EPOXIDE REDUCTASE

PROCOAGS LONGER $T_{1/2}$
2, 7, 9, 10

ACQUIRED THROMBOPHILIA
VIRCHOW'S = HYPERCOAGUABILITY
STASIS
ENDOTHELIAL INJURY

THROMBOPHILIA
— CANCER
— PROTEINS

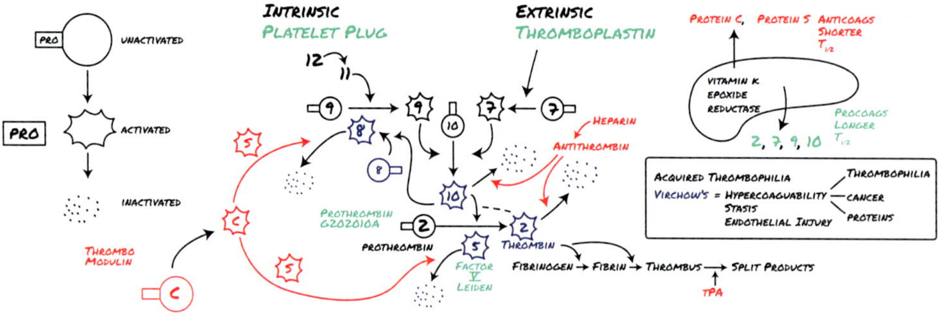

△ FACTOR FACTOR V LEIDEN A → G @ 506 ARG → GLN
PROTHROMBIN G20210A 3 UTR, ↑ PRODUCTION

DEFICIENCY ENZYME

PROTEIN C DEF — SKIN NECROSIS
PROTEIN S DEF — WARFARIN

ANTITHROMBIN DEF Ø △ PTT HEPARIN
TX DVT, ØDX

PLATELET ARTERIAL CLOTS CVA, CAD, PVD	HEART CHAMBERS AORTA ANTI-COAGULATIONS	VENOUS FACTOR THROMBUS DVT / PE
PLATELETS WHITE THROMBI (CLOT)	POST-MORTEM Ø LINES	FIBRIN VEINS RED THROMBUS
ANTI-PLATELETS		ANTI COAG

Clotting Pharmacology

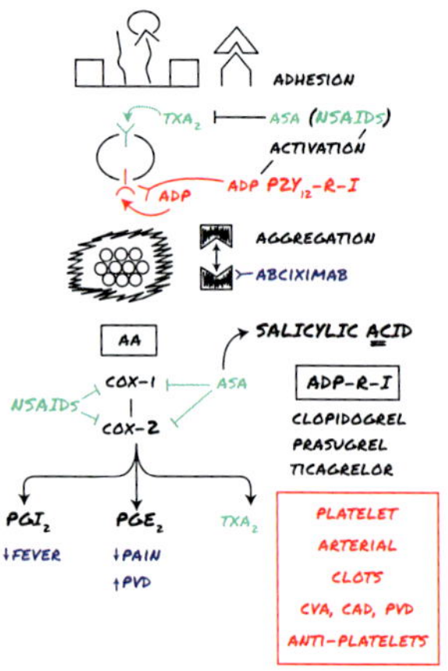

ADHESION

TXA₂ — ASA (NSAIDS)
ACTIVATION
ADP ADP P2Y₁₂-R-I
AGGREGATION
ABCIXIMAB

SALICYLIC ACID

AA

COX-1 — ASA
NSAIDS
COX-2

ADP-R-I
CLOPIDOGREL
PRASUGREL
TICAGRELOR

PGI₂ PGE₂ TXA₂
↓FEVER ↑PAIN
↑PVD

PLATELET
ARTERIAL
CLOTS
CVA, CAD, PVD
ANTI-PLATELETS

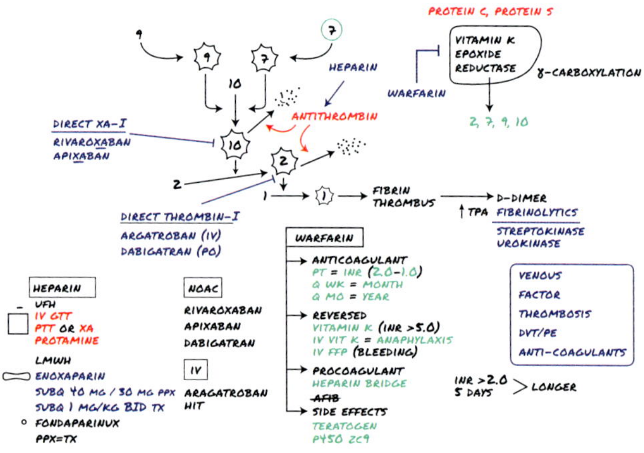

9
10
9 7
7

HEPARIN
ANTITHROMBIN

DIRECT XA-I
RIVAROXABAN
APIXABAN

10
2
2

WARFARIN

PROTEIN C, PROTEIN S
VITAMIN K EPOXIDE REDUCTASE
γ-CARBOXYLATION
2, 7, 9, 10

DIRECT THROMBIN-I
ARGATROBAN (IV)
DABIGATRAN (PO)

1 FIBRIN THROMBUS

D-DIMER
↑ TPA FIBRINOLYTICS
STREPTOKINASE
UROKINASE

HEPARIN
UFH
IV GTT
PTT OR XA
PROTAMINE

LMWH
ENOXAPARIN
SUBQ 40 MG / 30 MG PPX
SUBQ 1 MG/KG BID TX
○ FONDAPARINUX
PPX=TX

NOAC
RIVAROXABAN
APIXABAN
DABIGATRAN

IV
ARGATROBAN
HIT

WARFARIN
— ANTICOAGULANT
  PT = INR (2.0-1.0)
  Q WK = MONTH
  Q MO = YEAR
— REVERSED
  VITAMIN K (INR >5.0)
  IV VIT K = ANAPHYLAXIS
  IV FFP (BLEEDING)
— PROCOAGULANT
  HEPARIN BRIDGE
  AFIB
— SIDE EFFECTS
  TERATOGEN
  P450 2C9

INR >2.0
5 DAYS } LONGER

VENOUS
FACTOR
THROMBOSIS
DVT/PE
ANTI-COAGULANTS

Hematology Oncology

Platelet Bleeding

OnlineMedEd

↑BT PLATELET BLEEDING SUPERFICIAL, MUCOCUTANEOUS

(B5) GLYC 1B · VWF

TXA₂ · FIBRINOGEN · ADP

GLYC2B/3A (GT)

CLOTTING CASCADE

FIBRIN · FIBRIN CLOTS · D-DIMER

PLATELET COUNT — Low / NORMAL

Low → PETECHIAE → THROMBOCYTOPENIA — SEQUESTRATION / CIRRHOSIS

DESTRUCTION: HIT ITP, DIC TTP
PRODUCTION: CIRRHOSIS, BM DZ, CA, MFS

DIC — FIBRIN CLOTS ACTIVATION 1° + 2°, BLEEDING THROMBOSIS SAS
↓HGB, SCHISTO
↓PLT
↑INR
↓FIBRINOGEN
↑D-DIMER
UNDERLYING DZ GIVE BACK

TTP — HYALINE CLOTS, ↓ADAMTS 13, ↓PROTINASE,↑VWF, VWF MULTIMERS, FAT RN
HGB SCHISTO,↓HGB
PLT
INR —
FIBRINOGEN —
D-DIMER —
PLASMA EXCHANGE PFF

HIT — IgG vs PF-4, BOUND TO HEPARIN → PLT ACTIVATE → 10-14 DAYS ↓>50%, ≥25,000 NEW THROMBOSIS → STOP HEPARIN, ARGATROBAN

ITP — IgG vs GLYC2B/3A, SPLENIC DESTRUCTION, AUTOIMMUNE/MALIGNANCY, 1°ITP: ACUTE, KIDS, 2°ITP: CHRONIC,♀
STEROIDS, IVIg = PLASMAPHERESIS, SPLENECTOMY, RITUXIMAB

NORMAL → **PLATELET DYSFXN**
B5 / GT / VWD — DRUGS / UREMIA

VWD — MC INHERITABLE BLEEDING DISEASE, AUTOSOMAL DOMINANT, MILD... ASX UNTIL... MAJOR HEMOSTATIC
↓VWF → ADHESIONS → FACTOR 8 (↑PTT)
RISTOCETIN COFACTOR ASSAY (⊖,↓)
DESMOPRESSIN

Factor Bleeding

↑PTT: HEMOPHILIA, HEPARIN, VWD, INHIBITORS
INTRINSIC 12 11 9 8 | EXTRINSIC 7
10 5 2 1
↑PT: VIT K DEFICIENCY, WARFARIN, CIRRHOSIS, INHIBITOR, HEMOPHILIA
↑PT/PTT: HEMOPHILIA, INHIBITORS, DIC, SEVERE

HEMATOMAS FACTOR BLEEDING HEMARTHROSIS
COAG → ↑PTT / ↑PT / ↑BOTH
INTRINSIC / COMMON OR SEVERE / EXTRINSIC
INHIBITOR, DEFICIENCY

HEMOPHILIA — A 8,XR / B 9,XR: GIVE THE FACTORS THEY DON'T HAVE... ONLY WHEN BLEEDING; C 11,AR

VITAMIN K DEF — VITAMIN K FAT-SOLUBLE VITAMIN (A, D, E, K)
LEAFY GREENS, PANCREATIC LIPASE, TERMINAL ILEUM, GUT BACTERIA, NEWBORNS
CHRONIC ALCOHOLICS, PROLONGED ICU, NPO, CHRONIC PANCREATITIS, CYSTIC FIBROSIS, CROHN'S
PT PTT → INR
C,S
VITAMIN K EPOXIDE REDU
IM VITAMIN K, 2,7,9,10

MIXING STUDY
? + = PT
∅ CORRECTION
⊕ CORRECTION

LABJITSU
1 HEPARIN, ↑PTT
2 XA-I, THROMBIN-I, ↑PT, ↑PTT, ↑BOTH, NEITHER
3 LUPUS ANTICOAGULANT DOES NOT CORRECT THROMBOSIS

Hematology Oncology

Introduction to Proliferation

OnlineMedEd

#5 PLASMA CELL — HSC (CD34+) — CLP, CMP

CLP: T-CELL BLASTS → T-CELL LYMPHOCYTES CD 3, 4, 8; B-CELL BLASTS → B-CELL LYMPHOCYTES CD 19-22; MONO BLASTS → MONO CYTES

CMP: MYELO BLASTS → NEUTROPHILS, BASOPHILS, EOSINOPHILS; ERYTHRO BLASTS → ERYTHRO CYTES (RBC) #2; MEGAKARYO BLASTS → THROMBO CYTES (PLT)

CANCER
INSIDIOUSLY
↓ LAP
BLASTS
⊕ HSM
⊕ T(9,22)

BLAST — PRO — MYELO — META MYELO — BAND — PMN
← LEFT SHIFT

(CHRONIC) ↑ PROLIFERATION
BLAST CRISIS
BURNS OUT MYELOFIBROSIS
DE-DIFFERENTIATION

LEUKEMOID RXN
SUDDENLY
↑ LAP
MIX
NO HSM
NO T(9,22)

HGB
WBC ✕ PLT

↑ NUMBER
LEUKOCYTOSIS, NEUTROPHILIA
POLYCYTHEMIA
THROMBOCYTOSIS

↓ NUMBER
LEUKOPENIA, NEUTROPENIA
ANEMIA
THROMBOCYTOPENIA

LYMPHOMA VS LEUKEMIA

LYMPHOMA #4 → LYMPHO CYTES → MASS
LEUKEMIA → WBC, IN BLOOD

B-CELL LYMPHOMA
NODES, EBV
HODGKIN'S VS NHLS
(CD15-CD30) (CD20)

T-CELL LYMPHOMAS
RETROVIRUSES
NOT NODES

-PLASMA CELLS-

ACUTE VS CHRONIC

ACUTE
POORLY DIFFERENTIATED
CROWD OUT MARROW
FEVER, ANEMIA, BONE PAIN
NORMAL WBC
BLOOD SMEAR = BLASTS

CHRONIC
WELL DIFFERENTIATED
PT ASX
↑↑ WBC_DIFFERENTIAL
BLOOD SMEAR = MATURE

CMP / CML

#3
A M L   C M L
27 67   47
(APL)
A L L   C L L
?   67

MECHANISMS

JAK/STAT

JAK JAK
STAT
NUCLEUS

Chr 14   TRANSLOCATION
EBV
	LYMPHOMA	LEUKEMIA
	T(8,14)	T(12,21) ALL
	T(11,14)	T(15,17) APL
	T(14,18)	T(9,22) CML
	T(11,18)	

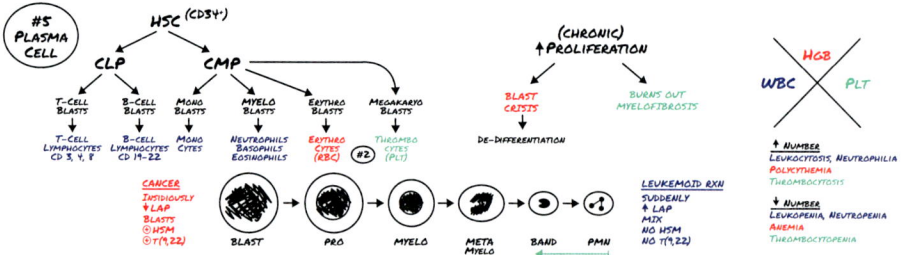

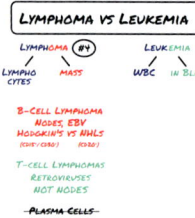

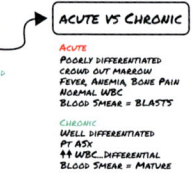

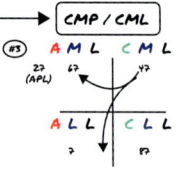

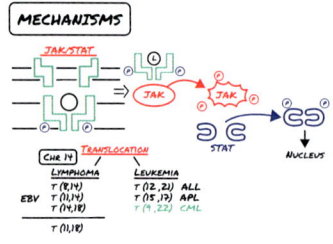

Myeloproliferation

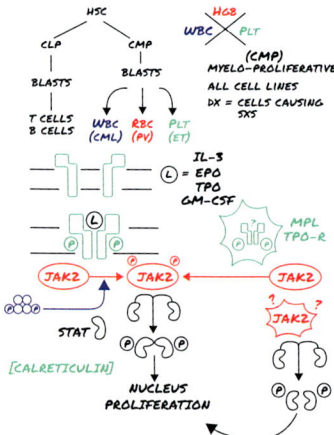

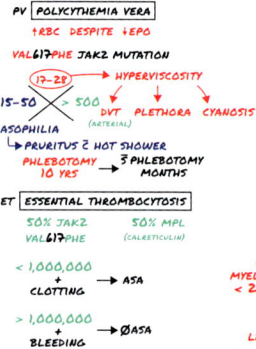

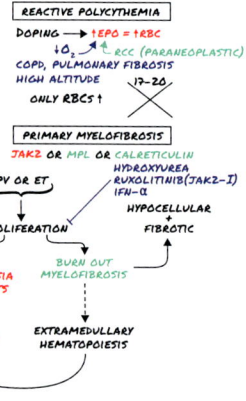

HSC — CLP, CMP

HGB
WBC ✕ PLT

(CMP)
MYELO-PROLIFERATIVE
ALL CELL LINES
DX = CELLS CAUSING SXS

CLP → BLASTS → T CELLS, B CELLS
CMP → BLASTS → WBC (CML), RBC (PV), PLT (ET)

IL-3
(L) = EPO
TPO
GM-CSF

JAK2 → JAK2 ← JAK2
MPL TPO-R
JAK2 ?
STAT
[CALRETICULIN]
NUCLEUS PROLIFERATION

POLYCYTHEMIA VERA
PV
↑ RBC DESPITE ↓ EPO
VAL617PHE JAK2 MUTATION

17-28 → HYPERVISCOSITY
15-50 > 500
DVT, PLETHORA, CYANOSIS (ARTERIAL)
BASOPHILIA
→ PRURITUS Ξ HOT SHOWER
PHLEBOTOMY 10 YRS → 3 PHLEBOTOMY MONTHS

ESSENTIAL THROMBOCYTOSIS
ET
50% JAK2   50% MPL
VAL617PHE   (CALRETICULIN)

< 1,000,000 + CLOTTING → ASA
> 1,000,000 + BLEEDING → ∅ ASA

REACTIVE POLYCYTHEMIA
DOPING → ↑ EPO → ↑ RBC
↓ O₂ ↗ RCC (PARANEOPLASTIC)
COPD, PULMONARY FIBROSIS
HIGH ALTITUDE
ONLY RBCs ↑   17-20

PRIMARY MYELOFIBROSIS
JAK2 OR MPL OR CALRETICULIN
HYDROXYUREA
RUXOLITINIB (JAK2-I)
IFN-α
PV OR ET
↑ PROLIFERATION → HYPOCELLULAR + FIBROTIC
CANCER MYELODYSPLASIA < 20% BLASTS
BURN OUT MYELOFIBROSIS
LEUKEMIA
EXTRAMEDULLARY HEMATOPOIESIS

OnlineMedEd

ACUTE LEUKEMIAS
- BM CROWDED OUT ⇒ ↓ CELL LINES
- BLASTS ON BLOOD SMEAR
- FLOW CYTOMETRY TO DISTINGUISH
- BM BX HAS > 20% BLASTS
  (< 20% MDS)

INFXN
ANEMIA
BLEEDING
HIGH FEVER
BONE PAIN
NRML WBC

CHRONIC LEUKEMIA
- INSIDIOUS
- ASX + ↑↑ WBC
- DIFFERENTIAL TO BLOOD SMEAR
- FLOW + BM BX DONE

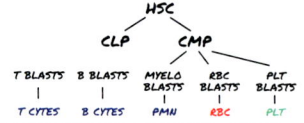

HSC — CLP, CMP
CLP: T BLASTS, B BLASTS
CMP: MYELO BLASTS, RBC BLASTS, PLT BLASTS
T CYTES, B CYTES, PMN, RBC, PLT

A M L
APL (27) = M3 VARIANT
T(15,17) RETINOIC ACID-R DEFECT
⊕ MPO ⊕ AUER RODS
↑[AUER] = ↑ CLOTTING CASCADE
DIC
ALL-TRANS RETINOIC ACID

AML 2/3 (67)
CML
ACCUMULATION OF MUTATIONS
BLAST CRISIS
FATAL, REFRACTORY

C M L (47)
T(9,22) = PHILADELPHIA CHR = BCR·ABL GENE FUSION
STABLE < 10% BLASTS
ACCELERATED 10%-20% BLASTS
6-12 MO   RAPID SPLENOMEGALY
BLAST CRISIS > 20% BLASTS
IMATINIB DASATINIB

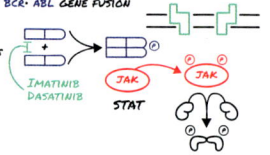

JAK   JAK
STAT

A L L (7)
B-CELL ALL
ONE MUTATION
T(12,21) = GOOD PROGNOSIS, MC CANCER CHILDHOOD
T(9,21) = POOR PROGNOSIS, BLAST CRISIS MULTIPLE MUTATIONS INTRATHECAL CHEMO PPX
T-CELL ALL   THYMIC MASS IN TEENAGERS

HSC 1/3
CLP   CD10 ⊕
TdT   TdT ⊕
T BLASTS   B BLASTS
T CYTES   B CYTES
CD 3, 4, 8   CD 19, 20, 21, 22

C L L (87)
ONLY A B-CELL VARIANT (CD5 ⊕)
↑↑↑ WBC + ASX = WAIT + WATCH
SMUDGE CELLS, MATURE LYMPHOCYTES
CLL → SCL → DLBCL ← FOLLICULAR LYMPHOMA
(BLOOD)   (NODE) RICHTER'S TRANSFORMATION   B-CELL CD5 ⊕

B CELL, NODES, EBV
HL
CD15/CD30', BUT ⊖ FOR LYMPHOCYTES EXPRESS ∅ IG
EBV → NF-KB = PROLIFERATION

CD40-L   CD15   CD30-L
CD40   CD30
Tₕ2   EOSINOPHILS
IL-5   IL-5
IL-10 → CD8

⊕ B SXS, CONTIGUOUSLY, IN NODES

ADULT T CELL
HLTV-1 = STI
JAPAN, WEST AFRICA, CARRIBEAN RAPIDLY FATAL

CD4' T HELPER

CUTANEOUS T CELL
SKIN
MYCOSES FUNGOIDES   T CELL SKIN
CEREBRIFORM
SEZARY   T CELL LEUKEMIA BLOOD

LYMPHADENOPATHY
FIXED, FIRM, HARD
PAINLESS, NONTENDER
CHRONIC

EXCISIONAL BIOPSY
⊕ RS   ∅
CD15'CD30'
HL   NHL

- A=DOXORUBICIN   RITUXIMAB (CD20)
  BLEOMYCIN   CYCLOPHOSPHAMIDE
- VINCRISTINE   H=DAUNORUBICIN
  DACARBAZINE   O=VINBLASTINE
  + XRT   PREDNISONE

STAGING
#LN   DIAPHRAGM
I   –   –
II   ≥ 2   SAME
III   ≥ 2   OPPOSITE/BOTH
IV   METASTATIC

"B SXS" = NIGHT SWEATS FEVER WEIGHT LOSS
⊕   ⊖
IIB   IIA

B CELL, NODES, EBV
NHL   CD20'

"78"   ① FOLLICULAR T(14,18)
BCL-2   ANTI-APOPTOSIS, ∅ PROLIFERATION
INDOLENT, RESISTANT, DO NOT TREAT
RITUXIMAB PALLIATIVE

BCL-6   ② DLBCL
MC NHL
LARGE B CELLS

✳   ③ BURKITT'S LYMPHOMA T(8,14)
"8"   KIDS, MITOTICALLY ACTIVE, EASY TO TREAT
C-MYC   CANCER CELLS, TINGIBLE MACROPHAGES
ⓐ ENDEMIC AFRICAN = MANDIBLE
ⓢ SPORADIC US   = PELVIS, EXTRANODAL

"11"   ④ MANTLE CELL T(11,14) CYCLIN D₁
CYCLIN   DISSEMINATED @ DX,
D₁   1/2 LEUKEMIA, HIGH MORTALITY
CD5 ⊕

⑤ MARGINAL ZONE T(1,18)   T(14,18)
H. PYLORI GALTOMA   T(11,14)
SJOGREN'S MALTOMA   T(8,14)

HEMATOGENOUSLY, ∅ B SXS, POOR PROGNOSIS

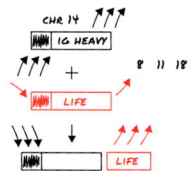

CHR 14
IG HEAVY
8 11 18
LIFE
LIFE

NOTES

Plasma Cell Dyscrasias

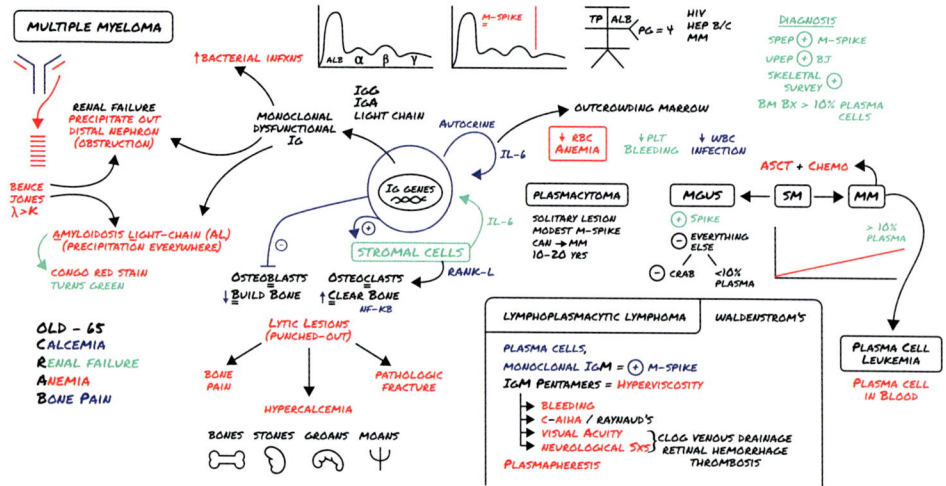

MULTIPLE MYELOMA

↑BACTERIAL INFXNS

RENAL FAILURE
PRECIPITATE OUT
DISTAL NEPHRON
(OBSTRUCTION)

MONOCLONAL
DYSFUNCTIONAL
IG

IGG
IGA
LIGHT CHAIN

AUTOCRINE

IG GENES

IL-6

STROMAL CELLS

BENCE
JONES
λ > K

AMYLOIDOSIS LIGHT-CHAIN (AL)
(PRECIPITATION EVERYWHERE)

CONGO RED STAIN
TURNS GREEN

OSTEOBLASTS
↓ BUILD BONE

OSTEOCLASTS
↑ CLEAR BONE
NF-KB

RANK-L

IL-6

ALB α β γ

M-SPIKE =

TP | ALB
PG = 4

HIV
HEP B/C
MM

OUTCROWDING MARROW

↓ RBC
ANEMIA

↓ PLT   ↓ WBC
BLEEDING INFECTION

PLASMACYTOMA

SOLITARY LESION
MODEST M-SPIKE
CAN → MM
10-20 YRS

MGUS → SM → MM

⊕ SPIKE

⊖ EVERYTHING
ELSE

⊖ CRAB   <10%
PLASMA

> 10%
PLASMA

DIAGNOSIS
SPEP ⊕ M-SPIKE
UPEP ⊕ BJ
SKELETAL ⊕
SURVEY
BM BX > 10% PLASMA
CELLS

ASCT + CHEMO

PLASMA CELL
LEUKEMIA

PLASMA CELL
IN BLOOD

OLD - 65
CALCEMIA
RENAL FAILURE
ANEMIA
BONE PAIN

LYTIC LESIONS
(PUNCHED-OUT)

BONE
PAIN

HYPERCALCEMIA

PATHOLOGIC
FRACTURE

BONES STONES GROANS MOANS

LYMPHOPLASMACYTIC LYMPHOMA   WALDENSTROM'S

PLASMA CELLS,
MONOCLONAL IGM = ⊕ M-SPIKE
IGM PENTAMERS = HYPERVISCOSITY

→ BLEEDING
→ C-AIHA / RAYNAUD'S
→ VISUAL ACUITY   } CLOG VENOUS DRAINAGE
→ NEUROLOGICAL SXS   RETINAL HEMORRHAGE
PLASMAPHERESIS   THROMBOSIS

Hematology Oncology

The Healthy Pituitary

OnlineMedEd

BRAIN **NEURAL ECTODERM**

SPHENOID

PHARYNGEAL ECTODERM — ROOF OF NASAL CAVITY

ME

TUBERALIS — INFUNDIBULUM
NERVOSA — DISTALIS
INTERMEDIA

SUPERIOR INFERIOR HYPOPHYSEAL ARTERIES
HYPOPHYSEAL PORTAL VEIN
POST / ANT
PEPTIDE HORMONES FENESTRATED CAPILLARIES
HYPOPHYSEAL VEINS
ADH
OXYTOCIN
REPRO

HYPOTHAL → HYPO HORMONE → ANTERIOR PITUITARY → AP HORMONE → EFFECTOR → HORMONE

NEURONS → SS / GHRH → SOMATO-TROPES → GH → LIVER → IGF-1

NEURONS → DOPAMINE (ON) → LACTO-TROPES → PRL → BREAST MILK / MILK

NEURONS → CRH → CORTICO-TROPES → ACTH → CORTISOL
STEROID HORMONES (ALDOSTERONE) CYTOPLASMIC-R

NEURONS → GNRH → GONADO-TROPES → FSH/LH → GONADS → SEX

NEURONS → TRH → THYRO-TROPE → TSH → THYROID → T4/T3
VITAMIN D NUCLEAR-R RXR

PEPTIDE HORMONES
2ND MESSENGERS
Gi — AC ← Gs
cAMP PKA CREB
Gq — IP3 DAG Ca2+ PKC
RTK — JAK STAT / BRAF + MAP KINASE / RET RAS PI3 KINASE AKT PTEN

The Unhealthy Anterior Pituitary

NEURAL — ADENOMA
MONOCLONAL NOT PREMALIGNANT
(+) HORMONE = FUNCTIONING
GH : GNAS = Gs ON
PRL : PIT-1
SXS OF HORMONE EXCESS
MICROADENOMAS < 1 CM
(-) HORMONE = HYPOFUNCTIONING
STRUCTURAL SXS
BITEMPORAL HEMIANOPSIA
MACROADENOMA ≥ 1 CM

PRL
ANTIPSYCHOTIC ESTROGEN (PREGNANCY) ⊥ TRH
HYPOTHAL
ON DOPAMINE ⊣ LACTROPES OMA
PRL
OVARIES ♀ AMENORRHEA + GALACTORRHEA
♂ ↓ LIBIDO
PT : ♂ MICRO + SXS PRL / ♀ MACRO + STRUCTURAL
DX : UPT, TSH, PROLACTIN → MRI
TX : CABERGOLINE >> BROMOCRIPTINE RESECTION + RADIATION

CHRONIC/INSIDIOUS
TUMOR — GH, FSH/LH, PRL
INFILTRATIVE — ACTH
AUTOIMMUNE — TSH
(INSULIN) VASOPRESSIN STIM TEST

ACUTE/CATASTROPHIC
INFECTION / INFARCTION / HEMORRHAGE / RESECTION — GIVE THEM WHAT THEY DON'T HAVE
LETHARGY, ↓BP COMA DEATH
SHEEHAN'S — POST PARTUM INFARCTION INABILITY TO LACTATE
APOPLEXY — PRE-EXISTING ADENOMA HEMORRHAGE

GH-OMA
HYPOTHALAMUS — SS — GHRH / GHRELIN
SOMATOTROPES
AC → cAMP → PKA
KETOGENESIS GLYCOGENOLYSIS GLUCONEOGENESIS FA OXIDATION
GH = PULSATILE RTK JAK/STAT CATABOLISM
FA MOBILIZATION TG SYNTHESIS
SKEL MUSCLE — ANABOLISM / ADIPOCYTES / HEPATOCYTES
IGF-1 RTK JAK/STAT (SUSTAINED) / IGF-1 / LINEAR GROWTH
BONES PATHOLOGIC GROWTH
TOO MUCH : ADULTS — ACROMEGALY / PEDS — GIGANTISM
HANDS TEETH SKULL — OTHER BONES : RINGS, HAT, GAPS; OTHER ORGANS : DJA CHF, HSM, ETC. ↑GH : HTN, DM, HLD, OBESITY
LONG BONES GROW = HEIGHT OTHER BONES GROW OTHER ORGANS — PROPORTIONALLY LARGE
DX : IGF-1 (GH) → GLUCOSE SUPPRESSION TEST (GH) → MRI
TX : SURGERY → OCTREOTIDE, PEG-VISO-MANT
TOO LITTLE : CONSTITUTIONAL GROWTH DELAY / BONE AGE
LARON SYNDROME GH-R DEF SHORT STATURE + SMALL, PROPORTIONATE VS ACHONDROPLASIA SHORT STATURE + NRML EVERYTHING

120 © 2021 OnlineMedEd

Endocrine

VOLUME = ALDOSTERONE = NaCL

MAP = CO X ↑SVR

↑HR X SV

↓PL X ↑CONT

TONICITY = ADH = WATER

P   C

PLASMA CELLS   HYPO-OSMOLAR   SWELLING

↓Na → ↓Sosm

P   C

HYPEROSMOLAR   SHRINKAGE

↑Na → ↑Sosm

RENIN → ALDO

ON

ENaC

H₂O

AQUAPORIN

ON   OFF

$U_{Na} < 10$ $U_{Na} > 20$ ALDO

$V_{OSM} > 300$ (800) $V_{OSM} < 300$ (100)   ADH

S_{OSM}
U_{Na}
U_{OSM}

VOLUME NORMAL

X CENTRAL ADH

X PLASMA CONCENTRATED

URINE DILUTE

DI

X CENTRAL ADH → DDAVP

CVA/TBI

X NEPHROGENIC
ADH-R
LITHIUM → STOP MEDICATION

V_{OSM}
800   RESTRICT H₂O   PP   CENTRAL
ADH
100   NEPHROGENIC
TIME

ADENOMA   SIADH

X BLOOD DILUTE

VOLUME NORMAL

DILUTE BLOOD

URINE CONCENTRATED   VOLUME LOSS   CONCENTRATED URINE
DEMECLOCYCLINE
-VAPTANS

HYPONA

X ← Sosm → X

↓(< 280)

HYPOOSMOLAR HYPONA

⊕ PHYSICAL   VOL STATUS   ⊕ HISTORY

OVERLOAD   EUVOLEMIC   VOL DEPLETE
DIURESIS   RTA
ADDISON
THYROID
SIADH   VOLUME

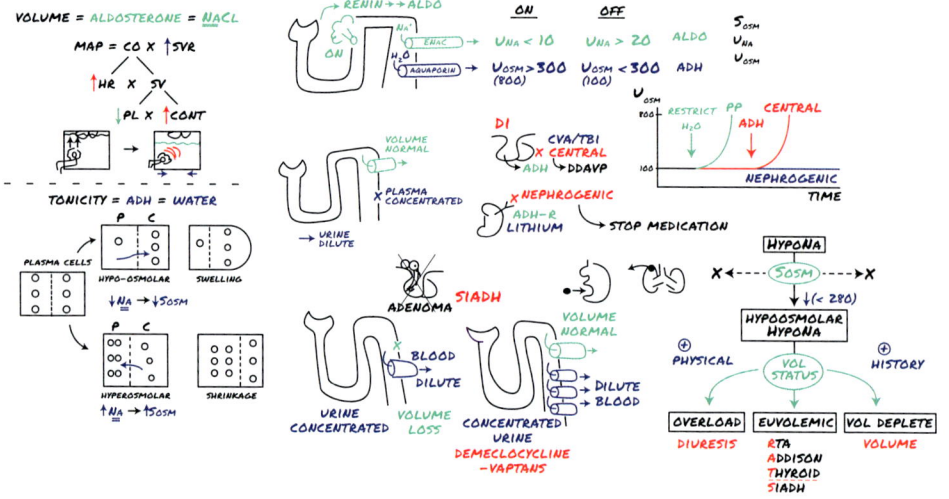

The Healthy Adrenal

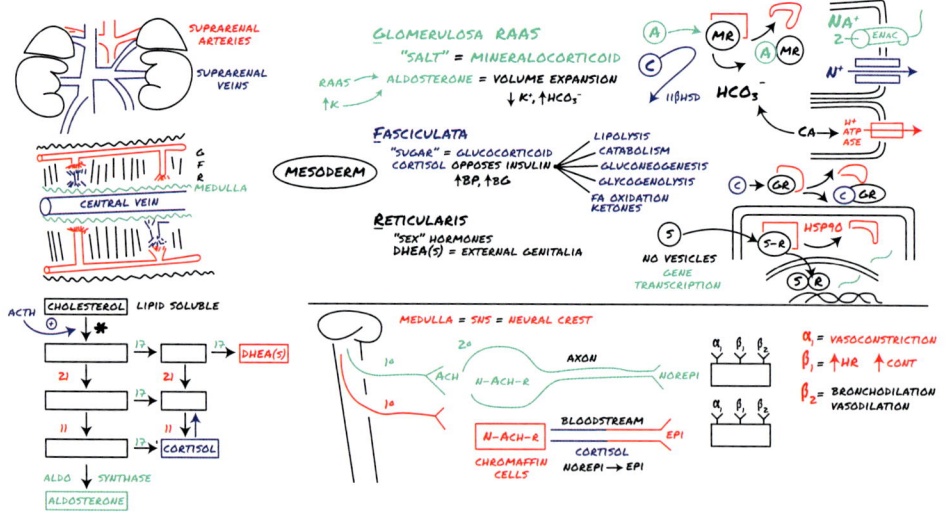

SUPRARENAL ARTERIES

SUPRARENAL VEINS

G
F
R
MEDULLA

CENTRAL VEIN

ACTH CHOLESTEROL LIPID SOLUBLE

1)
2)   2)   17   DHEA(S)
11   11   12
CORTISOL

ALDO SYNTHASE

ALDOSTERONE

GLOMERULOSA RAAS
"SALT" = MINERALOCORTICOID
RAAS → ALDOSTERONE = VOLUME EXPANSION
↓K⁺, ↑HCO₃⁻
↑K

FASCICULATA
"SUGAR" = GLUCOCORTICOID
CORTISOL OPPOSES INSULIN
↑BP, ↑BG

MESODERM

LIPOLYSIS
CATABOLISM
GLUCONEOGENESIS
GLYCOGENOLYSIS
FA OXIDATION
KETONES

RETICULARIS
"SEX" HORMONES
DHEA(S) = EXTERNAL GENITALIA

NO VESICLES
GENE TRANSCRIPTION

A → MR
C   A MR

11βHSD   HCO₃⁻

NA⁺
2 ← ENaC

N⁺

H⁺
ATP
ASE

CA →

C → GR   C GR

S   5-R   HSP90

5 R

MEDULLA = SNS = NEURAL CREST

2°

1°   ACH   N-ACH-R   AXON   NOREPI

1°

N-ACH-R
CHROMAFFIN CELLS   BLOODSTREAM
CORTISOL
NOREPI → EPI   EPI

α₁ β₁ β₂

α₁ β₁ β₂

α₁ = VASOCONSTRICTION
β₁ = ↑HR ↑CONT
β₂ = BRONCHODILATION
VASODILATION

Endocrine

Cortisol

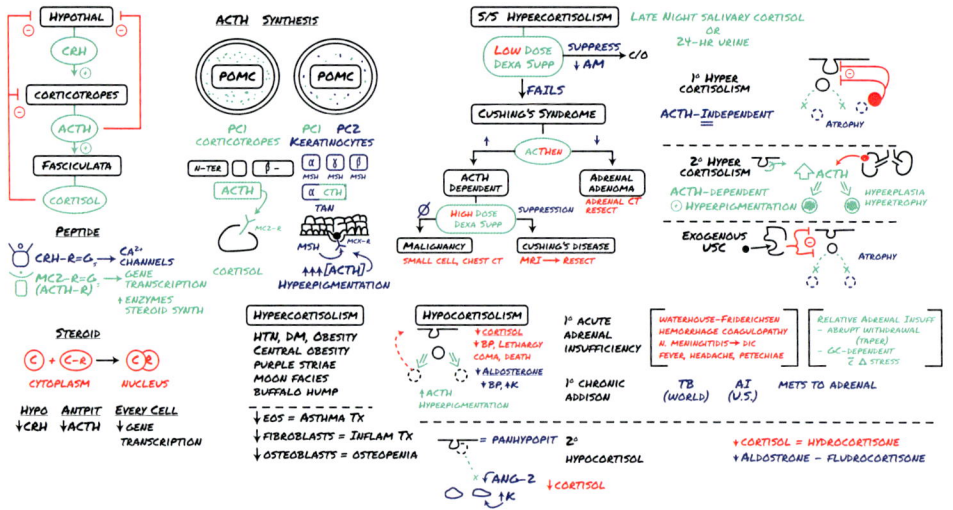

Aldosterone

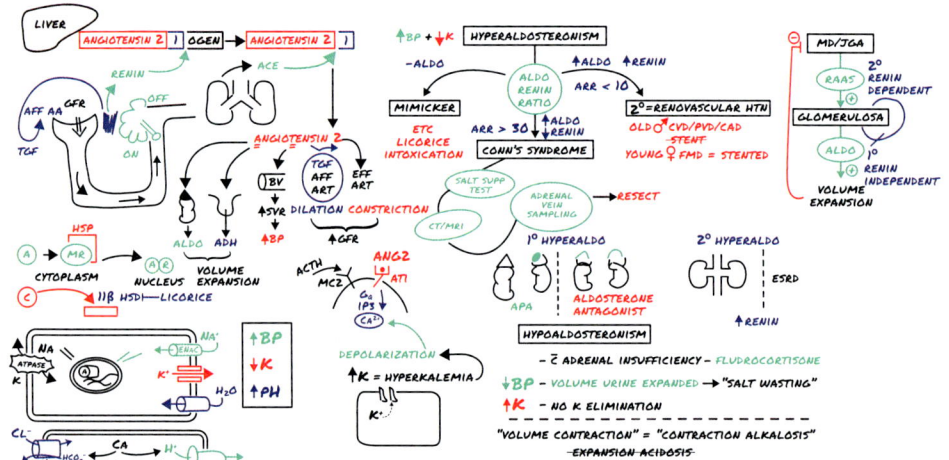

Endocrine

PHEOCHROMOCYTOMA

PATH: ADRENAL MEDULLA RET
(NOR)EPINEPHRINE

↓

(NOR)METANEPHRINE

↓

VMA

PT: **P**AROXYSMS
PALPITATIONS – β₁
PRESSURE – α₁
PAIN = HEADACHE
PALLOR
PERSPIRATION – α₁

SKIN HYPERPIGMENTATION

DX: ⊕ ATTACK SERUM CATECHOLAMINES
⊖ ATTACK 24-HR METANEPHRINE, VMA

↓

IMAGING: CT ADRENAL ⊖ ⟶ MIBG

TX: α-BLOCKADE = PHENOXYBENZAMINE
β-BLOCKADE = ?
RESECTION

PARAGANGLIOMA = PHEO NOT IN ADRENAL
NFI

MEN

MEN1
MEN1
PITUITARY
PARATHYROID
PANCREAS

GENE
NEOPLASMS

MEN2A
RET
PHEO
MEDULLARY
THYROID
CARCINOMA

MEN2B
RET
PHEO
MEDULLARY
THYROID
CARCINOMA

PARATHYROID

MUCOSAL
GLIOMA

PT c̄ ONE
IN ONE GLAND
+
FAM HX OF OTHER-
DIFFERENT GLADS

CAH

CHOLESTEROL

⇧ ACTH →

↓

DHEA(S) +/_ DHEA +/_ ALDO

	DEFICIENCY	EXCESS	XX	XY	BP	K
2)	DHEA		AMBIG	–	↓	↑
11						
17	ALDOS		–	AMBIG	↑	↓

CORTISOL

ALDOSTERONE

ANATOMY/HISTO

SUPERIOR
SUPERIOR LARYNGEAL
PYRAMIDAL
R ISTHMUS L
PARATHYROID
INFERIOR THYROIDAL AA
RECURRENT LARYNGEAL

COLLOID
BM
FOLLICLE
FENESTRATED ENDOTHELIUM
– SIMPLE CUBOID EPITHELIUM
– FOLLICULAR CELLS = THYROID HORMONE
– COLLOID = STORAGE FORM THYROID HORMONE
TG-IODINATED TYROSINES
– PARAFOLLICULAR CELLS = C CELLS CALCITONIN

SYNTHESIS

IODIDE UPTAKE = NIS Na-I-SYMPORTER
I RELEASE = PENDRIN

THYROID PEROXIDASE = OXIDATION (I⁻)
(TPO) ORGANIFICATION (I⁻)
MEMBRANE-BOUND COUPLING

THYROGLOBULIN (TG) = REALLY BIG AA CHAIN
c̄ TYROSINES

TYROSINE MIT DIT
ALA
RT₃ T₃ T₄

RELEASE

① PINOCYTOSIS – MEMBRANE FLUIDITY
② MEGALIN = FAILSAFE, BYPASSES LYSOSOME
CLATHRIN-MEDIATED ENDOCYTOSIS
INTACT TG RELEASED
② ??? = RIGHT WAY
ENDOCYTOSIS → FUSION c̄ LYSOSOME
LIBERATING T₃ AND T₄ ⟹ RELEASED
MIT, DIT DEIODINATED ⟹ TYROSINE + IODIDE
AA, IODIDE RECYCLED

CIRCULATION

FREE T₄/T₃ < 1%
ALBUMIN
PROTEIN-BOUND TRANSTHYRETIN
THYROID BINDING GLOBULIN
ADDED
RESERVE USED
RESUPPLIED

IN CELLS

T₃/T₄ – NUCLEAR-R
POTENCY T₃ >> T₄
QUANTITY T₄ >> T₃

T₄ → T₃ DEIODINASE
RETINOIC ACID
T₃ + RXR RECEPTOR

① ↑ Na⁺-K⁺ ATPASE
↑ MITOCHONDRIA
↑ CELLULAR RESPIRATION
GENERATE HEAT
② METABOLISM = "FUTILE CYCLES"

PROTEIN SYNTHESIS
MYOCYTES
PROTEIN CATABOLISM
LIPOLYSIS
ADIPOCYTES
TG SYNTHESIS

AXIS

HYPO
⊖ TRH
↑⊕
⊖ ANT PIT
TRH-R Gq-IP3-Ca²⁺
VESICULAR FUSION
TSH
TSH-R Gs-AC-cAMP-PKA
↑ GENE + ↑ PROTEIN ACTIVITY
↑ "SYNTHESIS" ↑ "RELEASE"
⊕ T₃/T₄

OUTCOME = ⚡ SPARK

HYPER		HYPO
↑HR ↑CONT, AFIB	HEART	↓HR ↓CONT
↑MOTILITY = DIARRHEA	GUT	CONSTIPATION
INSOMNIA, INABILITY TO CONCENTRATE EMOTIONALLY LABILE	BRAIN	LETHARGIC, COMA MENTAL RETARDATION
OSTEOPENIA HYPERCALCEMIA	BONE	GROWTH RETARDATION (CATCH-UP)
HEAT INTOLERANT	TEMP	COLD INTOLERANT
WEIGHT LOSS VORACIOUS APPETITE	METAB	WEIGHT GAIN
↑DTR	NERVES	↓DTR

Endocrine

The Unhealthy Thyroid—Functional Disorders

GRAVES' DZ

PATH: TSH-r AB, TYPE 2 HSR
STIMULATING, NONDESTRUCTIVE
PT: DIFFUSE GOITER
EXOPHTHALMOS (FIBROBLAST)—STEROIDS
PRETIBIAL MYXEDEMA

DX: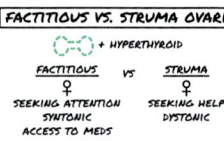

TOXIC ADENOMA

PATH: TSHR or GNAS = GoF
PT: SINGULAR NODULE

DX:

TOXIC MULTINODULAR GOITER

PATH: TSHR or GNAS = GoF, IODIDE DEF
PT: MULTIPLE NODULES, HX OF RECURRENT GOITER

DX:

FACTITIOUS VS. STRUMA OVARII

+ HYPERTHYROID

FACTITIOUS ♀	VS	STRUMA ♀
SEEKING ATTENTION		SEEKING HELP
SYNTONIC		DYSTONIC
ACCESS TO MEDS		

HYPERTHYROID

↑HR, AFIB
HEAT INTOLERANT
DIARRHEA
LOSS

↑
INSOMNIA
EMOTIONALLY LABILE

HYPOTHYROID

HR	TEMP	↓HR
	GI	COLD INTOLERANT
	WEIGHT	CONSTIPATION
	DTR	GAIN
	MENTATION	↓
		LETHARGIC

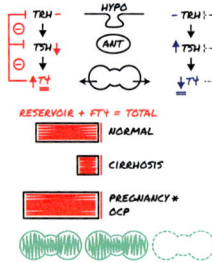

RESERVOIR + FT4 = TOTAL

- NORMAL
- CIRRHOSIS
- PREGNANCY *
  OCP

THYROIDITIS

HASHIMOTO'S ⊕TPO AB, ⊕TG AB LYMPHOCYTIC
TRANSIENT HYPER 2–6 WKS GERMINAL CENTERS
PERMANENT HYPOTHYROID → +HÜRTHLE
+FIBROSIS

SUBACUTE ⊕TPO AB, ⊕TG AB   LYMPHOCYTIC
(PAINLESS)   GERMINAL CENTERS

TRANSIENT HYPER 2–6 WKS → ⊕ PROGRESS
TRANSIENT HYPO 2–6 WKS↵   TO HASHIMOTO'S
[POSTPARTUM W/I 1 YR]

GRANULOMATOUS
(DE QUERVAIN) → VIRAL → HYPER → HYPO → RECOVER
PAINFUL   ILLNESS   2–6 WKS 2–6 WKS
                       (PAIN)   (PAIN)

VIRAL → MULTINUCLEATED → GRANULOMAS
AG   GIANT CELLS

REIDEL'S "ANAPLASTIC CARCINOMA" YOUNG

TREATMENT

- THIONAMIDES   PTU (1ST, THYROID   METHIMAZOLE (2ND, 3RD)
  INHIBIT TPO   STORM   TERATOGENIC
                 HEPATOTOXIC, 5 DEIODINASE
- RADIOACTIVE IODIDE (GRAVES, FOLLICULAR CARCINOMA)
- RESECTION (NODULES, CANCER, GRAVES)
- IODIDE = KI E HIGH DOSES = INHIBITORY
  (IV CONTRAST) SMALL DOSES = STIMULATORY
  LEVOTHYROXINE, 5X ⊕ TSH > 10

The Unhealthy Thyroid—Structural Disorders

NON-MALIGNANT

① ECTOPIC THYROID
MC = BASE OF TONGUE
∅ RISK CANCER, DYSFXN
LEAVE ALONE ⟶ RESECT

② THYROGLOSSAL DUCT CYST
CYST = MIDLINE, MOVES c̄ TONGUE

PHARYNGEAL   FOLLICULAR
EPITHELIUM   EPITHELIUM

③ GOITER = ↓↓↓. ♀ / GOITROGENS
RELATIVE IODIDE ↓ ♀ ↓T4/T3 → ↑TSH
DEFICIENCY

FOLLICLES ENLARGE, ↑COLLOID
↑TPO, ↑IODIDE UPTAKE, ↑REABSORPTION
T4/T3 NORMALIZE = TSH NORMALIZES
BIG THYROIDE = EUTHYROID STATE
REPEATED GOITER = MULTINODULAR

④ FOLLICULAR ADENOMA
TSHR, GNAS = HYPERFUNCTIONING
SMALL, CONTAINED BY CAPSULE
NOT PRE-MALIGNANT

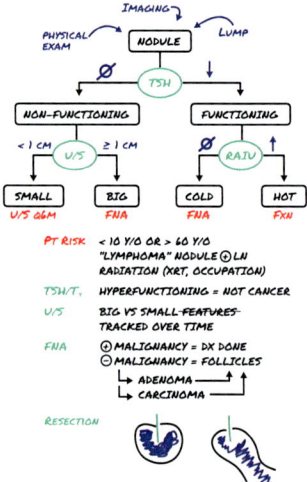

IMAGING

PHYSICAL   LUMP
EXAM ⟶ NODULE ⟵

∅
TSH

NON-FUNCTIONING   FUNCTIONING

< 1 CM | ≥ 1 CM   ∅ | RAIU
U/S

SMALL | BIG   COLD | HOT
U/S Q6M | FNA   FNA | Fxn

PT RISK   < 10 Y/O OR > 60 Y/O
           "LYMPHOMA" NODULE ⊕ LN
           RADIATION (XRT, OCCUPATION)
TSH/T.   HYPERFUNCTIONING = NOT CANCER
U/S   BIG VS SMALL FEATURES
           TRACKED OVER TIME
FNA   ⊕ MALIGNANCY = DX DONE
           ⊖ MALIGNANCY = FOLLICLES
           ↳ ADENOMA
           ↳ CARCINOMA

RESECTION

GENETICS

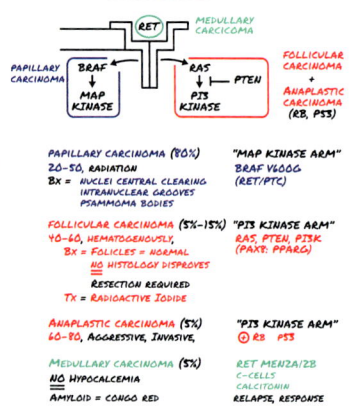

RET → MEDULLARY CARCINOMA
PAPILLARY CARCINOMA → BRAF → MAP KINASE
                      RAS → PI3 KINASE ← PTEN
                                          FOLLICULAR CARCINOMA
                                          + ANAPLASTIC CARCINOMA (RB, P53)

PAPILLARY CARCINOMA (80%)   "MAP KINASE ARM"
20–50, RADIATION   BRAF V600G
Bx = NUCLEI CENTRAL CLEARING   (RET/PTC)
     INTRANUCLEAR GROOVES
     PSAMMOMA BODIES

FOLLICULAR CARCINOMA (5%–15%)   "PI3 KINASE ARM"
40–60, HEMATOGENOUSLY,   RAS, PTEN, PI3K
Bx = FOLLICLES = NORMAL   (PAX8: PPARG)
     NO HISTOLOGY DISPROVES
     RESECTION REQUIRED
Tx = RADIOACTIVE IODIDE

ANAPLASTIC CARCINOMA (5%)   "PI3 KINASE ARM"
60–80, AGGRESSIVE, INVASIVE   ⊕ RB   P53

MEDULLARY CARCINOMA (5%)   RET MEN2A/2B
NO HYPOCALCEMIA   C-CELLS
AMYLOID = CONGO RED   CALCITONIN
                                 RELAPSE, RESPONSE

Endocrine

The Healthy Parathyroid

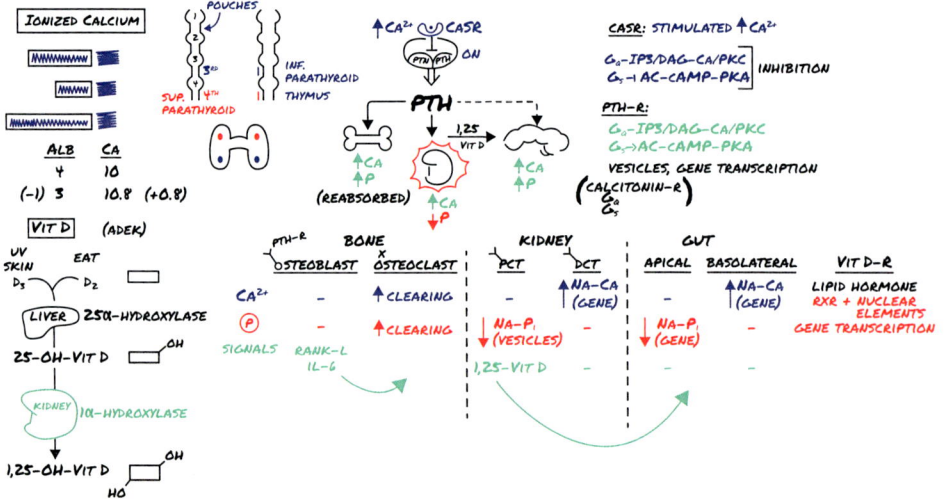

Unhealthy Parathyroid—Calcium Disorders

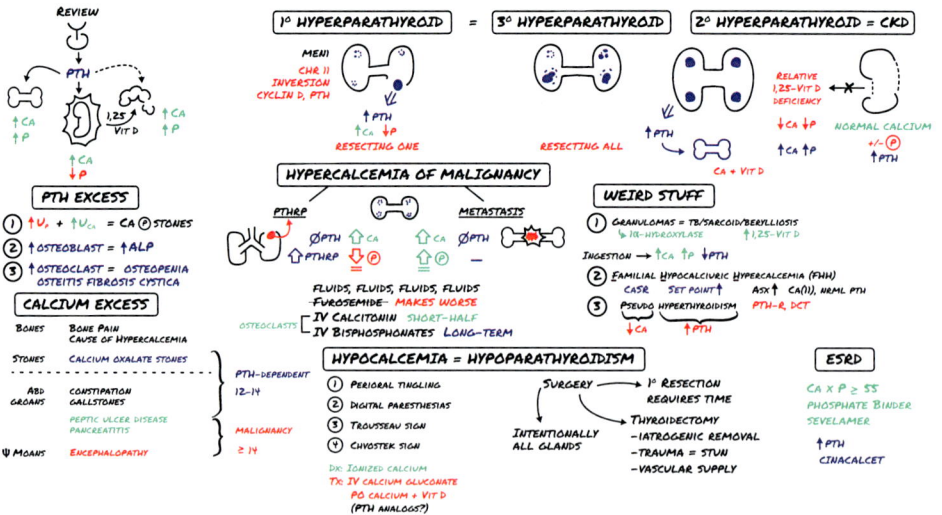

Endocrine

OnlineMedEd

NORMAL BONE

↳ **TYPES OF BONE**
LONG – EXTREMITIES
SHORT – HANDS/FEET
FLAT – STERNUM, SKULL
WEIRD – VERTEBRAE

↳ **LONG BONES**
CORTICAL
PERIOSTEUM
DIAPHYSIS – BM – ENDOSTEUM
METAPHYSIS – BV – TRABECULAR
EPIPHYSIS
CARTILAGE

↳ **HISTOLOGY**
– OSTEONS, OSTEONAL CANAL
– LACUNAE, CANALICULI, GAP JXNS
– CONCENTRIC/INTERSTITIAL LAMELLAE
– CEMENT LINES

↳ **MINERALIZATION**
– OSTEOID – ORGANIC – PROTEINS
  TYPE I COLLAGEN, PROTEINS, OSTEOCALCIN

– HYDROXYAPATITE $CA_{10}(P)_6OH_2$

– OSTEOBLASTS → OSTEOCLASTS
  OSTEOID   BONY MATRIX

ALKALINE   MATRIX
PHOSPHATASE   VESICLES

PLAYER/DIFFERENTIATION

"STROMAL" OB PRECURSOR OSTEOBLAST
ADIPOCYTES
CHONDROCYTES
BLC
ENDOTHELIAL FIBROBLAST   OSTEOCYTE OSTEOCLAST

OSTEOCLAST PRECURSORS
CFU
MACROPHAGE

INTERPLAY

BONE MARROW
OPG
RANK-L
IL-6
PTH-R
CSF

?
OPG
RANK-L
IL-6
CSF
← RANK-L
RANK
NF-KB

BONE
OPG
RANK-L
IL-6

?
OPG
RANK-L
IL-6

X

PROLIFERATE
DIFFERENTIATE
MATURATION

RANK IL-6
CALCITONIN
⊖

CA
H⁺ CL⁻
P
SEAL   SEAL
BONE   HCL

OSTEOBLASTS   **OSTEOCLASTS**

↳ BUILD BONE   CLEAR BONE
PTH-R   X
         RANK-L → RANK

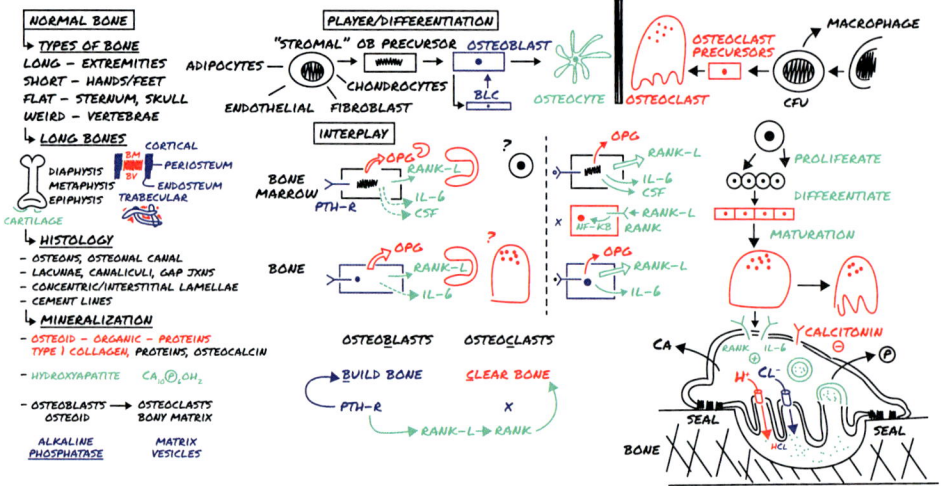

Unhealthy Bone

IN UTERO
WOVEN BONE – REMODELING – LAMELLAR
HAPHAZARD COLLAGEN – ALTERNATING COLLAGEN I
NO TENSILE STRENGTH – ↑ TENSILE STRENGTH

INTRAMEMBRANOUS OSSIFICATION
– FLAT BONES, VERTEBRAE
– NO CARTILAGE TEMPLATE
– MULTIPLE OSSIFICATION CENTERS

ENDOCHONDRAL OSSIFICATION
– CARTILAGE TEMPLATE
– OSTEOCYTES REPLACE CHONDROCYTES
– LONG BONES

VIT D DEFICIENCY
↳ RICKETS = KIDS
VIT D DEF. = 2° HPTH
↓CA ↓P   ↑CA ↑P
NORMAL CALCIUM @
THE COST OF BONES
① RADIOLUCENCY CORTEX
② WIDENING GROWTH PLATE
③ NON-AMBULATING
  –CRANIOTABES
  –FRONTAL BOSSING
  –RACHITIC ROSARY
  –PIGEON BREAST
④ AMBULATORY
  –BOW LEGS
  –LUMBAR LORDOSIS

↳ **OSTEOMALACIA = ADULTS**
2° HPTH → ↑ALP BONE PAIN
WEAKENED BONES = FX
DX: 25-VIT D (NRML CR)
TX: CA²⁺ + D₃ SUPP
1,25-VIT D

DIET OR UV LIGHT

OSTEOPOROSIS = OSTEOPENIA

30 60 90

PATH: OSTEOCLASTS OUTPACE
OSTEOBLASTS
NOT PTH-DRIVEN
TRABECULAR BONE
PT: HIPS = FX
VERTEBRAE = FX ↓HEIGHT
ASX-CA, P, PTH, ALP
SCREEN DEXA

EXERCISE – ↑IMPACT
WEIGHT LOW G AVOIDANCE
CA²⁺ + VIT D ⁻̄ MENOPAUSE
ESTROGEN → SERM
AVOID GLUCOCORTICOIDS
ETOH, TOBACCO

① BISPHOSPHONATES
  –DRONATE PO–GERD
  (ANNUALLY) IV=OSTEONECROSIS
② DANOSUMAB = OPG
  (ANNUALLY) IV=OSTEONECROSIS
③ TERIPARATIDE = PTH
  SQ RAPID ACTING

GROWTH
–CARTILAGE GROWTH PLATE
PROLIFERATION...CALCIFY...DIE
–OSTEOBLASTS USE CA²⁺
TO BUILD BONE
–REQUIRES CA²⁺
–REQUIRES VIT D

OSTEO-PETROSIS
PATH: AR LOF CA2 GENE
∅ CLEARING BONE
∅ BONE MARROW
∅ REMODEL
PT: PANCYTOPENIA EXTRAMEDULLARY
HEMATOPOIESIS HSM
WOVEN BONE = FX
OSSIFIED BONE XRAY
BEING BRIGHT WHITE
OVERGROWTH COMPRESSION
OF CRANIAL NERVES

OSTEOGENESIS IMPERFECTA
PATH: AD, COLLAGEN TYPE I
"MR. GLASS"
PT: BLUE SCLERA
FRACTURE EASILY
"ABUSE"
HEARING, DENTAL

ANCHONDROPLASIA
PATH: GOF FGF3,AD
LONG BONES TO NOT
GROW LONG
PT: SHORT STATURE
NRML INTELLECT
NRML HEAD
NRML LIFESPAN
NRML REPRODUCTION

PAGET'S
PATH: NF-KB ↑↑ OSTEOCLASTS
OCL BURNS OUT
OSTEOBLASTS BUILD BONE
3 REMODELING
PT: ≥ 70, ↑ALP, BONE PAIN
DX: X-RAY = SCLEROSIS
BX: MOSAIC PATTERN
PROMINENT CEMENT LINES
TX: BMT

Endocrine

OSTEOID OSTEOMA
DIAPHYSIS, M < 25, PAINFUL
OSTEOBLASTS = OSTEOID CORE
XR: RADIOLUCENT CORE $\bar{c}$
CORTICAL THICKENING
BX: OSTEOBLASTS PINK GOOP
TX: < 2 CM NSAIDS, NO SURGERY

OSTEOMA
GARDNER'S
COLON CANCER

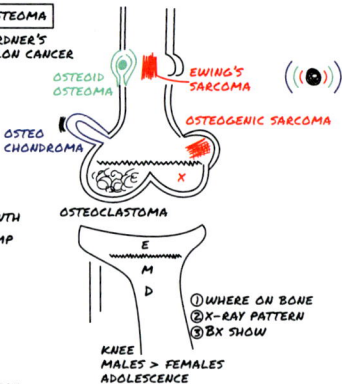

OSTEOBLASTOMA
> 2 CM
VERTEBRAE   } RESECT
UNRESPONSIVE NSAIDS

OSTEOCHONDROMA — MC BONY GROWTH
METAPHYSIS, M < 25, PAINFUL, BUMP
CONTINUOUS CORTEX, MEDULLA
CAPPED BY CARTILAGE
XR: CAULIFLOWER PROJECTION
TX: RESECT... CHONDROSARCOMA

OSTEOCLASTOMA
*EPIPHYSIS, AGE (20-40)
↑EXPRESSION RANK-L STROMAL
                    PROLIFERATION
                    +
OVERSTIMULATION ⇐ ACTIVATION
MULTINUCLEATED   LYTIC LESIONS
GIANT   ↑FX
OSTEOCLASTS

OSTEOID OSTEOMA
OSTEO CHONDROMA
EWING'S SARCOMA
OSTEOGENIC SARCOMA
OSTEOCLASTOMA

E
M
D
KNEE
MALES > FEMALES
ADOLESCENCE

① WHERE ON BONE
② X-RAY PATTERN
③ BX SHOW

EWING'S SARCOMA
DIAPHYSIS, MEDULLA, NEUROECTODERMAL
T11:22 (33)
PT: WHITE M < 15, BONE PAIN, FEVER, CYTOPENIAS
XR: ONION-SKIN APPEARANCE
BX: ANAPLASTIC RESEMBLE LYMPHOCYTES

OSTEOGENIC SARCOMA/OSTEOSARCOMA
1° = RB, ADOLESCENCE 2° = ELDERLY + PAGET'S
METAPHYSIS   + XRT
PT: BONE PAIN, FX, SURVEILLANCE
XR: SUNBURST CODMAN TRIANGLE
BX: EN BLOC RESECTION
    PLEOMORPHIC OSTEOBLASTS OSTEOGENIC
TX: PPX CHEMOTHERAPY   GOOP

CARTILAGE
CHONDROMA   CHONDROSARCOMA
BENIGN ⟶ MEDULLA ⟵ MALIGNANT
HANDS + FEET   SPINE/PELVIS

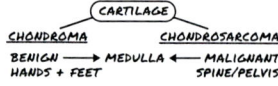

The Endocrine Pancreas

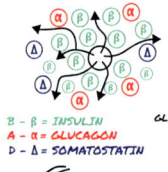

ISLETS
B - β = INSULIN
A - α = GLUCAGON
D - Δ = SOMATOSTATIN

PORTAL CIRCULATION
[INSULIN] OR [GLUCAGON]
TO HEPATOCYTES FIRST
(LARGEST SIGNAL)

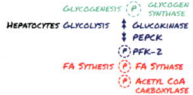

INSULIN   GLUCAGON
                    EPI
                    GH
                    CORTISOL

INSULIN SYNTHESIS
C
A   SIGNAL
B
PREPROINSULIN

A
B
PROINSULIN

A
B
INSULIN

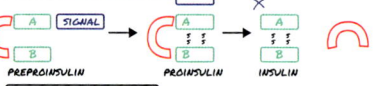

INSULIN RELEASE
GLUCOSE
GLUT2
K+
TCA
ETC
ATP
K
Ca²⁺
L-TYPE
Ca²⁺
CCK ACH   EPI GLUCAGON
Gq   Gs
IP3   AC
Ca²⁺   CAMP
           PKA
SS

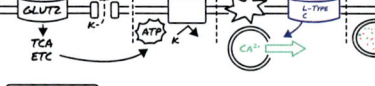

INSULIN R RTK⟶IRS
MYOCYTES
ADIPOCYTES
ALL OTHER
PI3 KINASE ⟶ GLUT4 VESICLES (EXERCISE)
AMINO ACID SYNTHESIS, TRIGLYCERIDE STORAGE, GLYCOGEN FORMATION
PROLIFERATION

GLUCONEOGENESIS GLYCOGEN SYNTHASE
HEPATOCYTES GLYCOLYSIS ↓ GLUCOKINASE
                        ↑ PEPCK
                        ↑ PFK-2
FA SYNTHESIS ↓ FA SYNTHASE
             ↑ ACETYL COA CARBOXYLASE

INSULINOMA
SYMPTOMATIC HYPOGLYCEMIA
① SXS = ↑HR, SWEATING, AMS/COMA
② ↓BG
③ REVERSES $\bar{c}$ DEXTROSE
DX: 72 HR FAST
    CT SCAN
TX: RESECTION

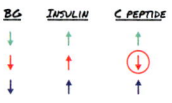

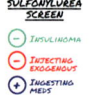

	BG	INSULIN	C PEPTIDE
	↓	↑	↑
	↓	↑	↓
	↓	↑	↑

SULFONYLUREA SCREEN
⊖ INSULINOMA
⊖ INJECTING EXOGENOUS
⊕ INGESTING MEDS

OTHEROMAS
-GLUCAGONOMA
MIGRATORY, NECROLYTIC ERYTHEMA
↑↑↑ GLUCAGON ⟶ CT

-SOMATOSTATINOMA
ACHLORHYDRIA FAT MALABSORPTION
GALLSTONES   STEATORRHEA
↑↑↑ SS ⟶ CT ⟶ SRS

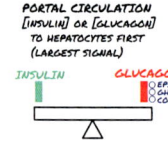

Endocrine

OnlineMedEd

TYPE I
PATH: AUTOIMMUNE DESTRUCTION
OF β-CELLS OF ISLETS
CD8 LYMPHOCYTES (TYPE 4)
⊕ AB-INSULIN, GAD, TP
NO β-CELLS = NO INSULIN
HISTO: "INSULITIS"
↓β-CELLS, ↓ ISLETS, LYMPHOCYTES
GENES: HLA-DR3/4
PT: CHILD/ADOLESCENT (LAG)
POLYDIPSIA, POLYURIA, WEIGHT LOSS
DKA
TX: INSULIN TO CONTROL BG

MYOCYTES | NO GROWTH CATABOLIC
ADIPOCYTES | NO GLUT4   ↑BG DIABETIC
    INSULIN HAPPENS
    TO ↓BG
↓GLUCAGON

200 300
  300 100 POLYURIA
  300   POLYDIPSIA
  100   VOLUME DEPLETE
            TOTAL BODY K↓
            WATER FOLLOWS OSM
            IV FLUIDS
            INSULIN ↓K   GIVE K

HEPATOCYTES ↑↑↑ GLUCONEOGENESIS
             ↑↑↑ GLYCOGENOLYSIS   INSULIN
             ↑↑↑ FA OXIDATION
EPI CORTISOL ↑↑↑ KETONES KETOACIDOSIS

TYPE II
PATH: INSULIN RESISTANCE
↑↑BG ↑INSULIN
↑↑↑ REGULATES   ↑↑↑ INSULIN
INSULIN-R   PRODUCED
                 -INSULIN
HISTO: AMYLIN AMYLOIDOSIS
GENES: STRONG! GENES?
PT: ASX ADULT, OBESE
SCREENING, BG, A1C
TX: NEXT LESSON

A1C
NRML < 5.7
PRE 5.7-6.3
DM ≥ 6.4

BG FASTING   GTT
NRM < 100   2 HR
PRE 100-124   < 140
DM ≥ 125   140-199
                    ≥ 200

NONENZYMATIC
GLYCATION

ADVANCED GLYCATION
END-PRODUCTS

MACROVASCULAR   MICROVASCULAR
ACCELERATED   LEAKY
ATHEROSCLEROSIS   CAPILLARIES
                              +VEGF
CAD PVD   CVD   NEPHROPATHY RETINOPATHY
(MI) (AMPUTATE) (CVA) (ESRD)   (BLIND)
                  [MICROALBUMINURIA] [RETINAL]

ENDO RAGE
      PROCOAGULANT
      DEPOSIT PROTEIN   ATHEROSCLEROSIS

MYOFIBROBLAST PROLIFERATION

BM
PROTEINS   LDL

↑BG
GLUT1 ↑[GLUCOSE]   GLUT5
(NEURONS)   (ENDO)
       ALDOSE
       REDUCTASE
       SORBITOL
       OSMOTIC SWELLING
NEURONS   LENS
NEUROPATHY   CATARACTS
[MONOFILAMENT]

↑BG

THICKENED BM

INTERCAPILLARY
GLOMERULOSCLEROSIS
            MESANGIAL
            SCLEROSIS

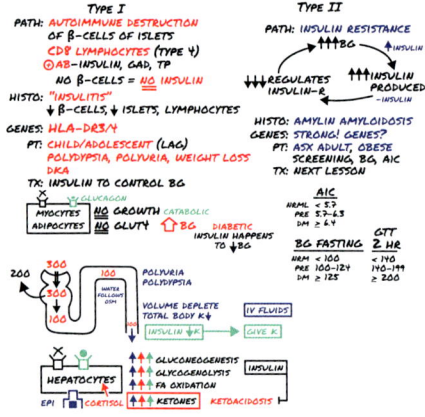

Diabetes Pharmacology

IF ↑INSULIN = HYPOGLYCEMIA, WEIGHT GAIN
INSULIN = GLUT4 MYOCYTES, ADIPOCYTES

INSULIN SENSITIZERS

* BIGUANIDES = METFORMIN
"MAGIC" DRUG   TIME-LIMITED DIARRHEA
NO HYPO   LACTIC ACIDOSIS
WEIGHT LOSS   RENAL FAILURE
DRUG #1   CONTRA: CKD

INSULIN RELEASE
                    ↑INSULIN
      MEDS   YES HYPO
                    WEIGHT GAIN
ATP   K+   K+   EXACERBATED IN AKI

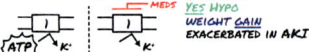

INCRETIN
        MIMIC/SUSTAIN INCRETINS
        PRIMES VERY LOW HYPO
   DPP4 PANCREAS
        ↑SATIETY WEIGHT LOSS
GLP-1   CAUSE PANCREATITIS + PANCREATIC
        CANCER

↓ TOTAL BODY GLUCOSE
- CELLS NOT METABOLISM
- INSULIN INDEPENDENT
- NO HYPO
- NO WEIGHT GAIN

-ROSI- PIO
TZD (-GLITASONE)
PPARγ = GLUT4
NO HYPO WEIGHT GAIN
CD = FLUID RETENTION
BM = OSTEOPENIA
     BLADDER CANCER

* SULFONYLUREAS
GLIMEPIRIDE
GLIPIZIDE
MEGLITINIDES

* GLP-1 ANALOGS (-ANATIDES)
EXENATIDE
INJECTABLE

DPP4-INHIBITORS (-GLIPTINS)
SAXAGLIPTIN
ORAL
DON'T WORK AT ALL?

* SGLT2-INHIBITORS (-GLIFLOZINS)
↓ PCT REABSORPTION GLUCOSE
GLUCOSURIA = DIURETICS
EUGLYCEMIC DKA IN TYPE 2
(CHEMO?)
SGLT2 VS. PLACEBO

α-GALACTOSIDASE-I
ACARBOSE
↑↑ ABSORPTION
B5
↓ DIGESTION
DIARRHEA, FLATULENCE
↑↑ PATIENT ADHERENCE

INSULINS

LONG-ACTING	RAPID-ACTING	MIXED
GLARGINE	ASPART	75-25
DETEMIR	LISPRO	70-30
DEGLUDEC	GLULISINE	50-50

NPH   REGULAR

STRATEGY

MIXED = "ONE MED," EASY, NO CLICKS, TWO STICKS
                    POOR CONTROL

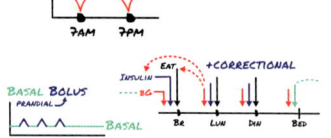

7AM 7PM

+CORRECTIONAL
Eat
INSULIN
-BG   Br Lun Din Bed

BASAL BOLUS
PRANDIAL
           BASAL

CARB COUNTING = B5, +CORRECTIONAL, CARB
                RATIO

"ARTIFICIAL PANCREAS"
SENSOR = CGM SQ
IV INFUSION = SQ PUMP
REGULAR

LAG

Endocrine

Introduction to Pulmonary

THORAX

1 – MANUBRIUM
2
3 } BODY
4
5-10-BODY
11 FREEFLOATING
12
POST
ANT

LINGULA L   R   L

ALVEOLAR 26-8YO

PARIETAL PLEURA
VISCERAL PLEURA

PLEURAL CAVITY MESOTHELIUM   "PLEURA"

EMBRYO

– ESOPHAGUS = ENDODERM

TRACHEA   1° BRONCHI
2° BRONCHI   WK 3-5 EMBRYONIC

3° BRONCHI   5-17 PSEUDO GLANDULAR
18 BRONCHO PULMONARY SEGMENTS

RESPIRATORY   TERMINAL   16-26 CANNALICULAR
BRONCHIOLES BRONCHIOLES
SACULAR 24-BIRTH

RESPIRATORY ZONE   CONDUCTING ZONE
GAS EXCHANGE   WARMS, HUMIDIFIES CLEANS AIR

O_2
CO_2

GOBLET   ASL   CILIATED COLUMNAR
MUCUS   SUBMUCOSAL GLANDS
MUCOCILIARY ESCALATOR

T/B

CARTILAGE   SMOOTH MUSCLE

TERMINAL BRONCHIOLES

RESPIRATORY BRONCHIOLES

MUCOSA EPITHELIUM BM LAMINA PROPRIA   SUBMUCOSA GLANDS LARGE VESSELS

H_2O x   x   x
CLARA CLUB

SURFACTANT

ALVEOLI

SEPTA =

TYPE 1 PNEUMOCYTES
TYPE 2 PNEUMOCYTES
ENDOTHELIAL
ALVEOLAR MACROPHAGE

Mechanics and Regulation of Respiration

MOVEMENT OF AIR

0   -2   0

0   +2

ELASTIC RECOIL

CHEST WALL OPENS
ALVEOLI COLLAPSE = ELASTIN
STRONGER WHEN STRETCHED

DYNAMIC COMPRESSION

SURFACE TENSION, COMPLIANCE

HYDROPHOBIC TAILS
HYDROPHILIC
↓STRETCHED ↑COLLAPSED SURFACTANT
TYPE 2 PNEUMOCYTES
DI-PALMITOYL-PHOSPHATIDYL-CHOLINE

SURFACTANT PROPORTIONATELY SURFACE TENSION
OPPOSES
$C = \dfrac{\Delta V}{\Delta P}$ COLLAPSED ALVEOLI HARD TO OPEN

REGULATION

– CENTRAL CHEMORECEPTORS
↓PH = ↑ VENTILATION
↑PH = ↓ VENTILATION
H^+
CA CO_2
2^- H_2O
HCO_3^-
MEDULLA = CSF H^+
– PERIPHERAL CHEMORECEPTORS CO_2
BLOOD

MOVING AIR = MUSCLES

OPEN = ↓P = ↑v = INSPIRATION
DIAPHRAGM
EXTERNAL INTERCOSTAL
PEC MINOR
STERNOCLEIDO-MASTOID
ACCESSORY M.

CLOSE = ↓v = ↑P = EXPIRATION
INTERNAL INTERCOSTAL
ABD MUSCLES
QUADRATOS

AVEOLI ELASTIC RECOIL
ACCESSORY M. EXPIRATION

PLEURAL PRESSURES. RV

-5 CMH$_2$O
RV

ALVEOLI ↑v
PLEURAL ΔP
-7 CMH$_2$O

VOL
= ALVEOLI ΔV
CHEST Ø Δ WALL
P   = PLEURAL ΔP

RR   ↓O_2 = ↑ VENTILATION
12
20 40 60 80 100   400
CARTOID – GLOSSOPHARYNGEAL
AORTIC – VAGUS
– OUTPUT IN MEDULLA

DRG   12 B/MIN DIAPHRAGM
x
- - DIAPHRAGM - - Acc - - Acc - - -
Ins   Exp
DRG   VRG

Pulmonary

PARTIAL PRESSURE

TOTAL BAROMETRIC PRESSURE (760)
"OTHER"=N_2
FIO_2 21% (160)

5,000 M (380) (80)

760 WATER (47) CO_2 (40)

$PIO_2 = FIO_2$ (TOTAL−WATER)

$PIO_2 = 150$

P [ALV] O_2=DIFFUSION

DIFFUSION GAS

PE
COPD

$D = K \times SA \times [GRAD]$

EDEMA   FIBROSIS
150   0
O_2 40/100
40   47 CO_2 40/100

$PACO_2 = PACO_2$

P [ALVEOLAR]   DIFFUSION−LIMITED
CARBON MONOXIDE (DLCO)

P [ALV]   PERFUSION−LIMITED
NO, CO_2

O_2 DIFFUSION

$PAO_2 − PaO_2 =$ AA GRADIENT ⊕ ≥ 10

$PAO_2 = PIO_2 − \dfrac{PACO_2}{0.8}$

$100 = 150 − 50$

TO ALVEOLI / TO CAPILLARY
ALTITUDE / LUNG DZ
NEUROMUSCULAR
OHS SEDATION
⊖A−A   ⊕A−A

OXYGEN DELIVERY

$D_cO_2 = CO \times HGB \times \%$ SAT
HR × SV $PAO_2 + 20 = \%$SAT
PRE × CONT   77 → 97
57 → 77
+ (PaO_2 × 0.003)   (↓20) → 100

HGB

CARBON DIOXIDE

① BICARBONATE (60%)
CARBONIC ANHYDRASE
$CO_2 + H_2O \rightleftharpoons H^+ + HCO_3^-$ Cl^-
(BOHR) H^+HB   DEOXY HGB   ↑AFFINITY H^+
↓AFFINITY O_2
H^+ DEOXY HGB

② CARBAMINO HGB (30%)
(HALDANE) CO_2 HB   DEOXY HGB   ↑AFF CO_2
↓AFF O_2
CO_2 DEOXY HGB

③ $P_V CO_2$ (10%)

ALVEOLAR VENTILATION

MV = RR × TV   ↑MV ↓CO_2

AV = RR × (TV − DSV)
350   500   150

ET TUBE

⊕ AERATED
⊖ PERFUSED

Pleural Lung Diseases

AUS   MEDIUM Δ = ↓SOUND
MORE SOLID = ↑SOUND

PER   MORE = DULL   MORE = RESONANT
SOLID   AIR

① PLEURAL EFFUSION
MEDIUM Δ=↓SOUND
SOLID = DULL
② PNEUMOTHORAX
MEDIUM Δ=↓SOUND
AIR = RESONANCE
③ CONSOLIDATION
MORE SOLID = ↑SOUNDS
SOLID = DULLNESS
④ PULMONARY EDEMA = CRACKLES
⑤ OBSTRUCTION
EXPIRATION = WHEEZE
INSPIRATION = STRIDOR

PULMONARY EDEMA

$J = K (H − O)$
INFLAM   CLOT
INFXN   CANCER
CANCER   COMPRESSION   "OSI"
CUTS   CIRRHOSIS
CIRRHOSIS   NEPHROSIS
GASTROSIS

ALI   vs   CHF

① CARDIOGENIC
TRANSUDATE = ↓PROTEIN ↓CELLS
HYDROSTATIC   CAUSE, ↑PCWP
CHF S/S: DOE, PND, ORTHOP
JVD, PERIPHERAL, ↑BNP EDEMA
H/O CHF, ECHO
HEMOSIDERIN−LADEN

② NONCARDIOGENIC
EXUDATIVE ↑PROTEIN −/−/−
↑CELLS
ALI=ARDS=DAD=HYALINE MEMBRANES

⊖OVERLOAD, ⊖H/O CHF
SEPTIC SHOCK   SIRS
PANCREATITIS
TRALI   VASODILATION
PMN, MACRO, FIBRO
COLLAGEN ← HM

PLEURAL EFFUSION

CHEST WALL v.   GRAVITY
LYMPHATICS

TRANSUDATE = H, O
EXUDATIVE = K, CA, INFXN

EFFUSION
LOCULATED   XRAY U/S   SIMPLE
THORACOSTOMY   THORACENTESIS
THORACOTOMY
*CHF DIVERSE

② HEMOTHORAX
PENETRATING OR BLUNT (RIB FX)
THORACOSTOMY
BRISK = SURGERY SLOW=
③ CHYLOTHORAX
LYMPHATIC OBSTRUCTION
MILKY WHITE (LIPID)
④ PARAPNEUMONIC EFFUSION
PNEUMONIA + EFFUSION
↑↑↑PMN,+/− ORGANISM
SURGERY

AIR

0CM
−7CM
−5CM

100% O_2 THORACOSTOMY

SIMPLE   LARGE   TENSION
SMALL   SIMPLE   PNEUMO

"PNEUMO" + HYPOTENSION
JVD
TRACHEAL DEVIATION
NEEDLE DECOMPRESSION

Pulmonary

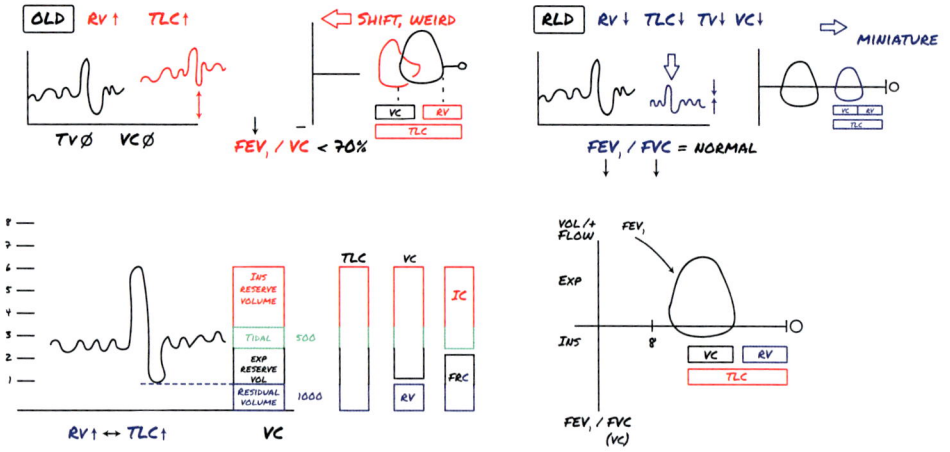

OLD RV↑ TLC↑

⟸ SHIFT, WEIRD

Tv∅ VC∅

↓ FEV₁ / VC < 70%

VC | RV
TLC

RLD RV↓ TLC↓ TV↓ VC↓

⟹ MINIATURE

FEV₁ / FVC = NORMAL
  ↓   ↓

VC | RV
TLC

8 —
7 —
6 —
5 —
4 —
3 —
2 —
1 —

INS RESERVE VOLUME
TIDAL 500
EXP RESERVE VOL
RESIDUAL VOLUME 1000

TLC   VC

IC

RV

FRC

RV↑ ⟷ TLC↑   VC

VOL /+ FLOW   FEV₁
EXP

INS   8

VC | RV
TLC

FEV₁ / FVC (vc)

Obstructive Lung Disease

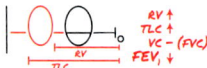

RV↑
TLC↑
VC – (FVC)
FEV₁ ↓

RV / TLC

FEV/FVC ↓< 70%
FEV₁ 80% → 20%

↑CO₂

CHRONIC BRONCHITIS

PATH: LARGE AIRWAYS
PT: SMOKER, OLD

• CHRONIC PRODUCTIVE COUGH
  > 3 MO IN > 2 YRS, HYPOXEMIA

• CYANOSIS, PULM HTN, Ⓡ CHF
  PERIPHERAL EDEMA, JVD
  "BLUE BLOATERS"

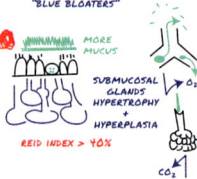

MORE MUCUS

SUBMUCOSAL GLANDS HYPERTROPHY + HYPERPLASIA

↓ O₂

REID INDEX > 40%

CO₂ ↓

EMPHYSEMA

PATH: ALVEOLI, LOSS OF ELASTIN/SEPTA
PT: SMOKER

PROLONGED EXPIRATORY, PURSED LIPS
INTERCOSTAL HYPERTROPHY
CACHEXIA, ↑AP DIAMETER
XR = HYPERINFLATION
CHRONIC CO₂ RETAINERS
  – PH ↑ PCO₂ ↑BICARB

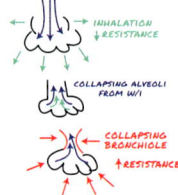

← INHALATION → ↓ RESISTANCE

COLLAPSING ALVEOLI FROM W/I

COLLAPSING BRONCHIOLE
↑RESISTANCE

CENTRIACINAR SMOKING APICES

① INFLAMMATION
  DEBRIS → PMN
  ↑PROTEASES

② ANTIPROTEASE
  A1AT DEFICIENCY
  CIRRHOSIS, EMPHYSEMA

③ APOPTOSIS?
  VEGF – ENDOTHELIAL
    ↳RTP3QI – MTOR
  NRF–2 – OXIDANT
    STRESS GENES

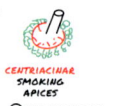

LOWER LOBES

PANACINAR A1AT DEF

IRREVERSIBLE
OLD SMOKERS

REVERSIBLE
YOUNG DON'T SMOKE

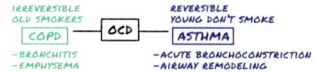

COPD ⟷ OCD ⟷ **ASTHMA**

–BRONCHITIS
–EMPHYSEMA

–ACUTE BRONCHOCONSTRICTION
–AIRWAY REMODELING

ASTHMA

PATH: REVERSIBLE CONSTRICTION
  TYPE / HSR = IgE, MAST, EO
PT: YOUNG, NORMAL BETWEEN ATTACKS
  WHEEZE DYSPNEA, COUGH
  ↑CO₂, ↓O₂

REVERSE ⊂ BETA–AGONISTS
INDUCE METHACHOLINE

AIRWAY REMODELING
– SUBMUCOSAL HYPERTROPHY +
  HYPERPLASIA
– GOBLET HYPERPLASIA
– SMOOTH MUSCLE HYPERTROPHY
– SUB BASEMENT FIBROSIS

① EARLY PHASE=CONSTRICTION

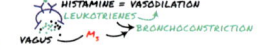

HISTAMINE = VASODILATION
LEUKOTRIENES
VAGUS — M₃ → BRONCHOCONSTRICTION

② LATE PHASE = MUCUS ↓

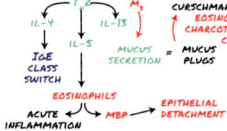

T 2   M₃
IL–4 ↙ ↘ IL–13
IgE   MUCUS
CLASS   SECRETION
SWITCH

= MUCUS PLUGS

SPUTUM
CURSCHMANN SPIRALS
EOSINOPHILS
CHARCOT LEYDEN CRYSTALS

EOSINOPHILS

ACUTE INFLAMMATION → MBP → EPITHELIAL DETACHMENT

Pulmonary

Obstructive Lung Disease Pharmacology

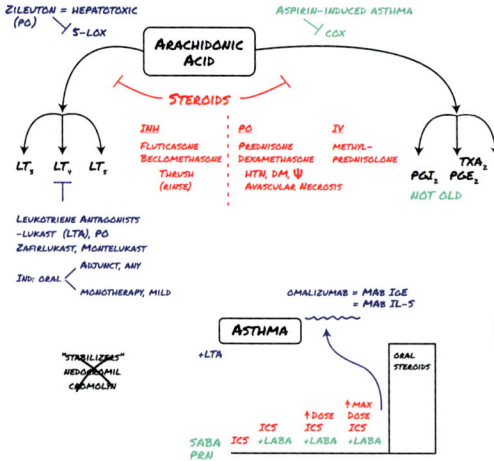

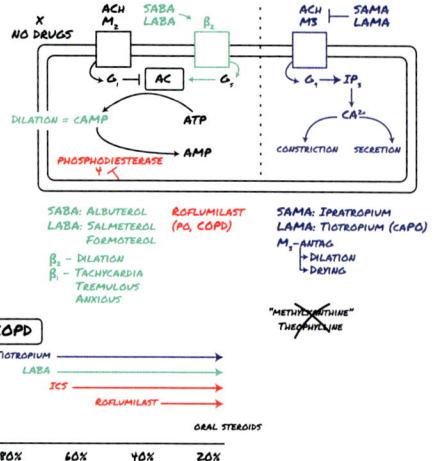

ZILEUTON = HEPATOTOXIC (PO)
5-LOX

ASPIRIN-INDUCED ASTHMA
COX

ARACHIDONIC ACID

STEROIDS

INH	PO	IV
FLUTICASONE	PREDNISONE	METHYL-
BECLOMETHASONE	DEXAMETHASONE	PREDNISOLONE
THRUSH	HTN, DM, ↓	
(RINSE)	AVASCULAR NECROSIS	

LT₃ LT₄ LT₅
PGI₂ PGE₂ TXA₂
NOT OLD

LEUKOTRIENE ANTAGONISTS
-LUKAST (LTA), PO
ZAFIRLUKAST, MONTELUKAST
ADJUNCT, ANY
IND: ORAL
MONOTHERAPY, MILD

"STABILIZERS"
NEDOCROMIL
CROMOLYN

OMALIZUMAB = MAB IgE = MAB IL-5

ASTHMA
+LTA
ORAL STEROIDS

SABA ICS ICS ↑DOSE ICS ↑MAX DOSE ICS
PRN +LABA +LABA +LABA

X NO DRUGS

ACH M₂ ⊣ SABA LABA β₂

ACH M₃ ⊣ SAMA LAMA

Gᵢ — AC — Gₛ

Gᵢ → IP₃
Ca²⁺

DILATION = cAMP ATP

PHOSPHODIESTERASE AMP

CONSTRICTION SECRETION

SABA: ALBUTEROL
LABA: SALMETEROL FORMOTEROL

ROFLUMILAST (PO, COPD)

SAMA: IPRATROPIUM
LAMA: TIOTROPIUM (CAPO)
M₃-ANTAG
DILATION
DRYING

β₂ – DILATION
β₁ – TACHYCARDIA
TREMULOUS
ANXIOUS

"METHYLXANTHINE"
THEOPHYLLINE

COPD
TIOTROPIUM
LABA
ICS
ROFLUMILAST
ORAL STEROIDS

80% 60% 40% 20%

Restrictive Lung Disease

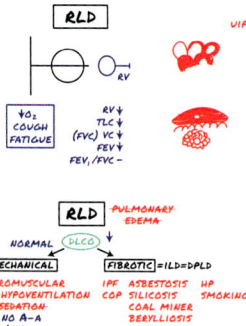

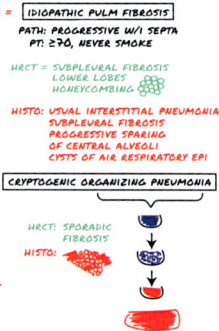

RLD

RV

+O₂
COUGH
FATIGUE

RV ↓
TLC ↓
(FVC) VC ↓
FEV ↓
FEV₁/FVC –

RLD — PULMONARY EDEMA

NORMAL DLCO ↓

MECHANICAL   FIBROTIC =ILD=DPLD

NEUROMUSCULAR IPF ASBESTOSIS HP
OBESITY-HYPOVENTILATION COP SILICOSIS SMOKING
SEDATION COAL MINER
NO A-A BERYLLIOSIS
↑CO₂

VIP = IDIOPATHIC PULM FIBROSIS
PATH: PROGRESSIVE W/I SEPTA
PT: ≥70, NEVER SMOKE

HRCT = SUBPLEURAL FIBROSIS
LOWER LOBES
HONEYCOMBING

HISTO: USUAL INTERSTITIAL PNEUMONIA
SUBPLEURAL FIBROSIS
PROGRESSIVE SPARING
OF CENTRAL ALVEOLI
CYSTS OF AIR RESPIRATORY EPI

CRYPTOGENIC ORGANIZING PNEUMONIA

HRCT: SPORADIC FIBROSIS
HISTO:

DUST	RISK	LOBE/HISTO	OTHER
ASBESTOSIS	CONSTRUCTION -PLUMBER -ELECTRICIAN SHIPYARDS	LOWER LOBES SUBPLEURAL FIBROSIS	ADENOCARCINOMA MESOTHELIOMA FERRIGINOUS BODIES
		PLEURAL PLAQUE	
SILICOSIS (MC)	CONCRETE BUILDING DEMOLISHING CLEANING (SAND-BLASTING)	UPPER LOBES FIBROTIC NODULES EGG SHELL CALCIFICATION	TB
COAL MINER'S (CARBON)	COAL EXPOSURE -MINERS -SOOT CITY	UPPER LOBES BLACK LUNG NODULES-PINK COLLAGEN + BLACK CARBON EMPHYSEMA = ALVEOLI SEPTA	ANTHRACOSIS (NOT DPLD)
BERYLLIOSIS	AEROSPACE	UPPER LUNGS	–

144

Pulmonary

Pneumonia

PNA MECHANISMS
1. IMPAIRED COUGH/↑ASPIRATION
   - SEDATED
   - NEUROMUSCULAR DZ
   - COMA
2. MUCOCILARY ESCALATOR
   - CIGARETTES
   - POST-VIRAL
   - GENETICS
3. OBSTRUCTION
4. IMMUNODEFICIENCY

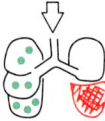

BRONCHIOLAR / DIFFUSE CONSOLIDATION
LOBAR PNA / LOCALIZED CONSOLIDATION

① **CONGESTION 1D**
- BACTERIA ARRIVE
- MACROPHAGES SOUND ALARM INFLAMMATION
- VENOUS STASIS, ARTERIAL DILATION
- FLOODING ALVEOLUS

② **RED HEPATIZATION 3D**
- FIBRIN EXUDATE
- NEUTROPHILS ARRIVE, DUMP
- RBCS COME TOO

CONSOLIDATION / NOT AERATED HEPATIZATION — RED COLOR / FOCUS-LUNG

③ **GRAY HEPATIZATION 4-7D**
- FIBRIN EXUDATE
- NEUTROPHILS WON, MACROPHAGES ENGULF BACTERIA, NEUTROPHILS
- RBCS CLEANED UP

CONSOLIDATION UNCHANGED, GREY

④ **RESOLUTION + ORGANIZATION**

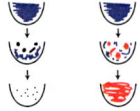

NECROTIZING = ABSCESS

PATH: ANAEROBES LOVE TO BE FLOODED
PT: HIGH FEVER, AIR-FLUID
HISTO: LIQUEFACTIVE NECROSIS + PMNS
TX: CLINDAMYCIN

INTERSTITIAL PNA
- INTRACELLULAR PATHOGENS
  └ VIRUSES └ CHLAMYDIA
               └ MYCOPLASMA
- NO ALVEOLAR PATHOGENS
  NO ALVEOLAR EXUDATE
- LYMPHOCYTES + MACROPHAGES IN SEPTA
- PROTEINACIOUS MATRIX IN SEPTA
- SELF-RESOLVE, MILD

GUESS BUG

MC	STREP PNEUMO
COPD	HEMOPHILUS
ASPIRATION	KLEBSIELLA (ETOH)
POST-FLU	STAPH AUREUS
NECROTIZING	ANAEROBES

GUESS THE DRUG

"WALKING PNA" DOXYCYCLINE / AZITHROMYCIN

CAP: β-LACTAM + MACROLIDE
CEFTRIAXONE + AZITHRO
(MOXIFLOXACIN)

HCAP: MRSA + PSEUDOMONAS

VANCOMYCIN PIP-TAZO + CIPRO
LINEZOLID   CEFEPIME + "
            MEROPENEM + "

Lung Cancer

INCID   MORTAL
GENDER   LUNG
LUNG → COLON
COLON   GENDER

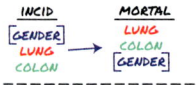

METS TO >> 1° LUNG CANCER
LUNG   (1 LESION)
(MULTIPLE)

SMOKING/GENES

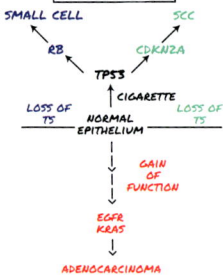

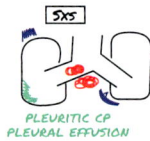

SMALL CELL   SCC
   RB   CDKN2A
       TP53
      CIGARETTE
LOSS OF NORMAL   LOSS OF
TS   EPITHELIUM   TS
         ↓
       GAIN OF FUNCTION
         ↓
       EGFR KRAS
         ↓
   ADENOCARCINOMA

Sxs

COUGH (75%)
HEMOPTYSIS (50%)
SVC SYNDROME
DIAPHRAGMATIC PARALYSIS
HOARSENESS
DYSPHAGIA

PLEURITIC CP
PLEURAL EFFUSION

55-80
30 PACKYR
<15 YRS QUIT
QIY

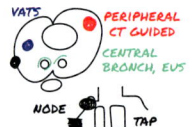

VATS
PERIPHERAL CT GUIDED
CENTRAL BRONCH, EUS

NODE   TAP

	CANCER	GENE	RISK	PARANEOPLASTIC	LOCATION	HISTOLOGY
EPI	ADENO(40%)	EGFR KRAS	♀ SMOKERS NONSMOKERS	–	PERIPHERAL	GLANDS MUCIN⊕
	SCC (30%)	TP53 CDKN2A	♂ SMOKERS	PTHrP	CENTRALLY	DESMOSOMES KERATIN WHORLS
NEURO ENDOCRINE	SMALL CELL (15%)	TP53 RB	SMOKERS	SIADH=↓NA ACTH=CUSHING'S LAMBERT-EATON	CENTRALLY	SMALL CELLS NUCLEUS SYNAPTOPHYSIN CHROMOGRANIN A
	LARGE CELL (10%)	–	–	–	–	ANAPLASTIC CYTOPLASM A LOT
	CARCINOID (5%)	–	–	CARCINOID SYNDROME	–	WELL ORGANIZED TRABECULAE LOW MITOTIC RATE
	MESOTHELIOMA	–	ASBESTOS	–	PLEURA	MESOTHELIUM

Pulmonary

Pulmonary Circulation

24/12 (MAP 15)
$P_vO_2 = 40$
$P_vCO_2 = 46$

$R = 5$ L/MIN
$L = 5$ L/MIN

$D = SA \times \dfrac{(GRAD)}{T}$

PUSH + PULL

↑PBF = ↓PVR

HYPOXIA

↓O_2 LUNGS VASOCONSTRICTION

120/80 (MAP=90)

CLOSE CAPILLARIES
OPEN ARTERIOLE
CLOSE ART
OPEN CAP

RV   VOL   TLC

EXERCISE
↑CO = HR × SV
RECRUITMENT   DILATION
↑SA
$\dfrac{V}{Q} \approx 1$

↑M_v = Tv × RR
↑A_v = ALVEOLAR VENTILATION
↑SA

REABSORPTION   P 90
FILTRATION
$J = k\,(P - \pi)$
L M S ART COP

$P_aO_2 = 80$
$P_aCO_2 = 80$

$\dfrac{\downarrow V}{\uparrow\uparrow Q}$

"ZONES" = GRAVITY

1   $\dfrac{\uparrow V}{\uparrow\uparrow Q}$
2
3

$P_A > P_a > P_v$ = COLLAPSED
$P_a > P_A > P_v$ = OPEN + NONCONDUCTING
$P_a > P_v > P_A$ = OPEN + CONDUCTING

DEAD SPACE
$M_v = RR \times T_v$
$A_v = RR \times (T_v - DS_v)$

500   150
300   150
150   150

Pulmonary Embolism

DVT

STASIS : IMMOBILITY
CHF
"LONG-DISTANCE-TRAVEL"

HYPERCOAG : ACTIVE MALIGNANCY
↑ESTROGEN, OCP, HRT
OBESITY ♀

ENDOTHELIAL DAMAGE : CATHETER

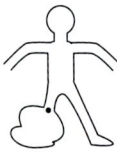

① DEEP VEINS
② DISTAL LE
③ Ⓤ > 3 CM CIRCUM
④ U/S COMPRESSION DOPPLER
RULE IN : U/S
RULE OUT : D-DIMER

Tx : STABILIZE = LMWH
MAINTENANCE = NOAC, WARFARIN
RESOLUTION = RECANALIZATION

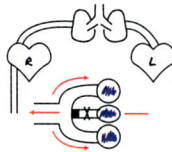

R   L

① V/Q MISMATCH
HYPOXEMIA → HYPER VENTILATION → RESP ALKALOSIS
TACHYCARDIA → ↑CO = V/Q ≈ 1

② ACUTE PULM HTN

ⓡ ♡ STRAIN
— BNP
— TROPONIN
— ECHO
$S_1Q_3T_3$

ⓛ ♡ FAILURE
JVD, HYPOTENSION

③ HEMORRHAGE
⊕ HEMOPTYSIS
⊕ PLEURITIC CP

④ INFARCT
DUAL BLOOD SUPPLY
WEDGE-SHAPED

	SX	Ⓡ STRAIN	SHOCK	TX
ASX	⊖	⊖	⊖	BRIDGE, NOAC
SX	⊕	⊖	⊖	LMWH → ORAL
SUBMASSIVE	⊕	⊕	⊖	HEPARIN IV
MASSIVE	⊕	⊕	⊕	TPA

CTEPH   PLUM HTN   THROMBECTOMY

V/Q SCAN   CTA

REQUIRES GOOD LUNGS   REQUIRES GOOD Cr

≤2	3-5	≥6
R/O   R/I

<4	≥4 YES

WELL'S CRITERIA : ZOMFG!?!?
3
⊕ DVT

1.5
IMMOBILE
SURGERY
H/O DVT
TACHYCARDIA

1
HEMOPTYSIS
MALIGNANCY

OTHER PE

① FAT
LONG BONE FX
1-3 DAYS ⊅
NEUROLOGIC, PETECHIAE

② AMNIOTIC
VAGINAL DELIVERY
DIC, SHOCK

③ AIR
NSG UPRIGHT
> 100 CC SX PE
NOVICE PROCEDURE

④ DECOMPRESSION
SCUBA DIVER
BENDS
CHOKER

⑤ SEPTIC
⊕ BLOOD CXS
MULTIPLE FOCI
SEPTIC ALREADY

Pulmonary

Pulmonary Hypertension

V - "OTHER"
V/Q, ANGIOGRAM

HIGH REZ CT
RLD
OLD PFT

PVR ↑
MEDIAL THICKENING
RV HYPERTROPHY
↑ PULM PRESSURE
ECHO: EPAP
↓ "STUFF"
RIGHT HEARTH CATH VASODILATOR
<5% → CCB ⊕
>95% → +/- BX

II ECHO

ANA, TSH, HIV, SCL-70...ETC.

IV
CTE PH
- HX DVT/PE
- V/Q SCAN ANGIOGRAPHY
  +
- THROMBECTOMY
- THROMBUS ⇄ RECANALIZED

III
HYPOXEMIC LUNG
- MEDIAL THICKENING + HYPERPLASIA
- OLD PFT
- RLD PDT, CT } O₂
- OSA/OHS SLEEP/MASK

II
LV DYSFXN
- PULMONARY VENOUS HTN
  ↳ VENOUS MEDIAL THICKENING
  ↳ ARTERIALIZATION
- CHF SXS, PULMONARY EDEMA
  ↳ HEMOSIDERIN MACROPHAGES
- ECHO
- TX=CHF

I
PULMONARY ARTERIAL HYPERTENSION
- → 2° PAH
- INTIMAL THICKENING
- FIBROBLAST PROLIFERATION
- COLLAGEN, COLLAPSES LUMEN
  ↳ IPAH
- PLEXIFORM LESIONS
- BMRP-2
- YOUNG ♀ 20-40
  DX ⊖
- BX = DX
  EPOPROSTENOL

LOUD S₂
JVD
PERIPHERAL EDEMA
DIASTOLIC DYSFXN

BOSENTAN
ORAL, HEPATOTOXIC
TERATOGENIC

SILDENAFIL TADALAFIL
PDE-5 INHIBITORR
ORAL, SAFE, ↑IUGR

PROSTACYCLIN INFUSED

ENDOTHELIN
↳ PROLIFERATION VASOCONSTRICTION

NO
GC ⟨ GTP
cGMP
VASODILATION
PDE-5

G₅ → AC-cAMP VASODILATION

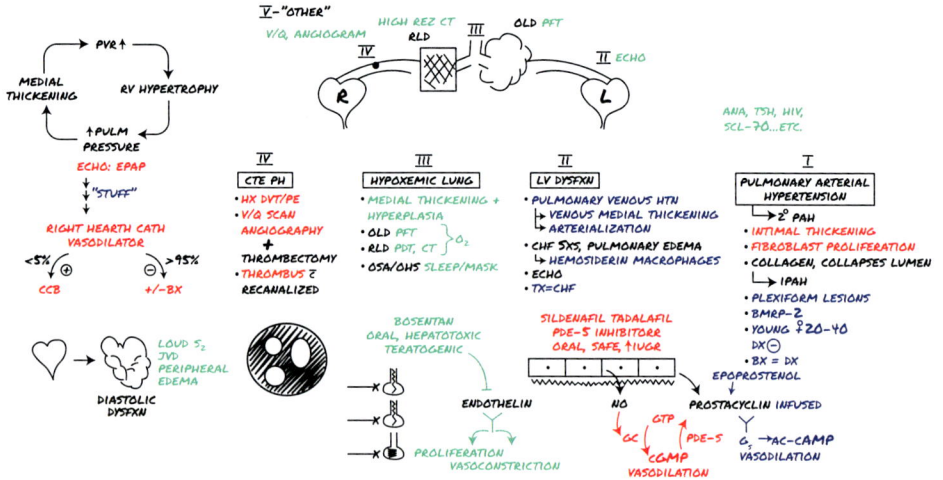

Ear Nose Throat Pathologies

RESPIRATORY
STREP PNEUMO
HEMOPHILUS, MORAXELLA

NASAL / SINUSES

↳ **VIRAL RHINOSINUSITIS**
ADENO -, RHINO -, CORONA VIRUS (36°C)
CLEAR RHINORRHEA, VIRAL SXS, NO FEVER
PRESSURE, ∓ PAIN/TENDERNESS
INFLAMED MUCOSA

↳ **BACTERIAL SINUSITIS**
ANTECEDENT VIRAL INFECTION IMPROVES...
PURULENT RHINORRHEA, FEVER
PAIN + TENDERNESS → MAXILLARY

↳ **ALLERGIC RHINITIS**
TYPE 1 HSR = IGE, MAST, EO
ASTHMA ALLERGIES ATOPY
NASAL POLYPS

↳ **CHOANAL ATRESIA**
Ⓑ ATRESIA = NEONATAL
BLUE WHEN FEEDING
PINK WHEN CRYING

SSCE = GROUP A STREP PYOGENES, STAPH AUREUS

NASOPHARYNX / OROPHARYNX

↳ **PHARYNGITIS**
VIRAL >> STREP
PSGN + RHEUMATIC ♡
ERYTHEMATOUS OROPHARYNX
ODYNOPHAGIA → EARS

⊖ Cough
Exudate
Nodes
Temp >100.4
0 < 13 + 1
R ≥ 45 - 1

↳ **PERITONSILLAR ABSCESS**
4-7YO, DROOLING, HIGH FEVER
HOT POTATO VOICE
UVULA DEVIATION
ABX + DRAINAGE

↳ **RETROPHARYNGEAL ABSCESS**
4-7YO, DROOLING, HIGH FEVER
HOT POTATO VOICE
NECK FLEXED + ANTERIOR LN
ABX + DRAINAGE → OR

↳ **OTITIS MEDIA**
EAR PAIN, PAINFUL SWALLOWING, FEVER
⊕ PNEUMATIC INSUFFLATION
FLUID, PUS, ETC.
EAR TUBES

↳ **NASOPHARYNGEAL CARCINOMA**
AFRICA EBV   NITROSAMINE SE ASIA

BOTH

LARYNX

↳ **CROUP** RSV
6 MO - 3 YO, STRIDOR
SEAL-BARK COUGH

↳ **EPIGLOTTITIS** HIB ⊢ VACCINE
4Y-7YO, DROOLING, HIGH FEVER
NECK EXTENSION
STRIDOR → OR

↳ VOCAL CORD LESIONS

SCC
ADENO

SQUAMOUS CELL CARCINOMA

VOCAL CORD NODULES
Ⓑ < 1CM
OVERUSE

PAPILLOMA
ⓥ < 1CM
HPV 6, 11

ⓥ > 1CM
HPV 16, 18
SMOKING

Pulmonary

OnlineMedEd

140 TRILLION SYNAPSES
86 MILLION NEURONS

NUCLEI +
    TRACTS

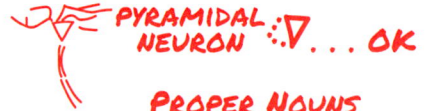

PYRAMIDAL
NEURON ∴∇ . . . OK

1 SECOND = 1000 MS
ACTION POTENTIAL
3-5 MS

ABSOLUTE REFRACTORY
PERIOD 1-2 MS

[5 + 2] MS MAX
IN 1 SECOND ≈ 140 APS

PROPER NOUNS

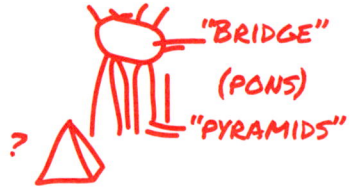

"BRIDGE"
(PONS)
"PYRAMIDS"

?

CONDUCTION VELOCITY
60 M/SECOND
196 FT/SECOND
34 DUSTYNS/SECOND

The Normal CNS—Cells, Fascicles, and Meninges

GREY VS. WHITE

GREY = NEURON CELLBODIES
+ GLIAL CELLS
WHITE = NEURON AXONS
+ GLIAL CELLS (MYELIN)

NEURONS

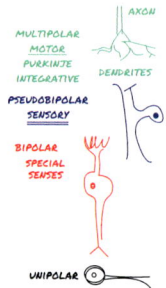

MULTIPOLAR
MOTOR
PURKINJE
INTEGRATIVE   AXON

PSEUDOBIPOLAR
SENSORY   DENDRITES

BIPOLAR
SPECIAL
SENSES

UNIPOLAR

PERIPHERAL NERVES CENTRAL FASCICLES

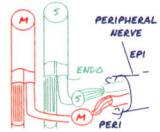

PERIPHERAL NERVE
EPI
ENDO
PERI

SUPPORT CELLS

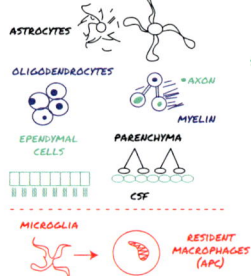

ASTROCYTES

OLIGODENDROCYTES
= AXON
MYELIN

EPENDYMAL CELLS
PARENCHYMA
CSF

MICROGLIA → RESIDENT MACROPHAGES (APC)

ASTROCYTES

① BLOOD-BRAIN BARRIER
 · ENDOTHELIAL TIGHT JUNCTIONS
 · ASTROCYTE FOOT PEDICLES
 · INTERLOCKING FEET

② MODULATE   SYNAPSES + NODES
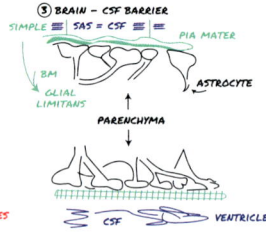
OR
SYNAPSE   NODE

SPATIAL BUFFERING (GAP JUNCTIONS)
SUB STRATE BUFFERING (K+, LACTATE, NT)

③ BRAIN - CSF BARRIER
SIMPLE ≡ SAS = CSF ≡ ≡   PIA MATER
BM
GLIAL LIMITANS   ASTROCYTE

PARENCHYMA

CSF   VENTRICLE

MENINGES

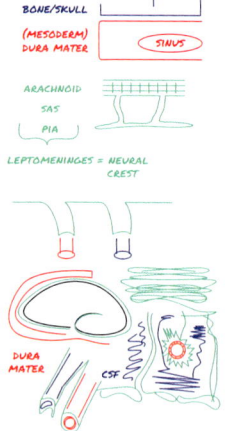

BONE/SKULL
(MESODERM) DURA MATER   SINUS

ARACHNOID
SAS
PIA

LEPTOMENINGES = NEURAL CREST

DURA MATER   CSF

NOTES

The Flow of CSF—Ventricles and Sinuses

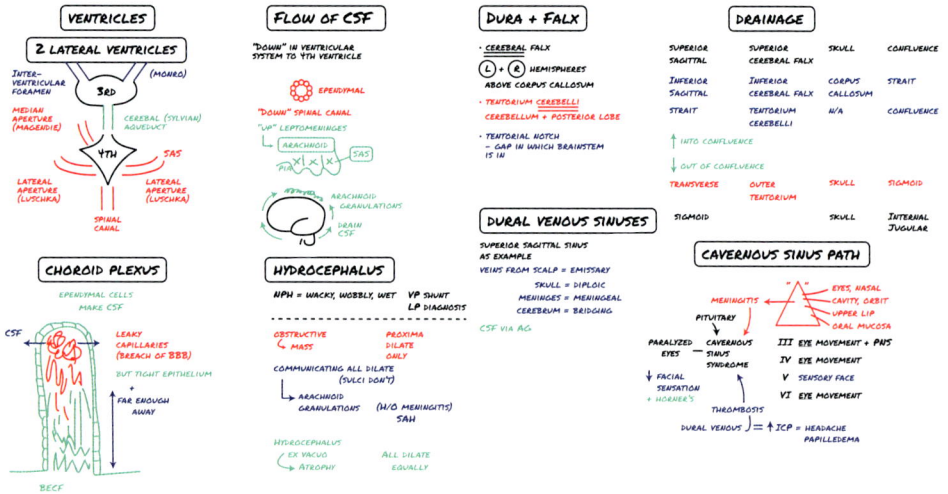

OnlineMedEd

VENTRICLES

2 LATERAL VENTRICLES

INTER-VENTRICULAR FORAMEN | (MONRO)
3RD
MEDIAN APERTURE (MAGENDIE) | CEREBAL (SYLVIAN) AQUEDUCT
4TH | SAS
LATERAL APERTURE (LUSCHKA) | LATERAL APERTURE (LUSCHKA)
SPINAL CANAL

CHOROID PLEXUS

EPENDYMAL CELLS MAKE CSF

CSF
- LEAKY CAPILLARIES (BREACH OF BBB) BUT TIGHT EPITHELIUM
- + FAR ENOUGH AWAY

BECF

FLOW OF CSF

"DOWN" IN VENTRICULAR SYSTEM TO 4TH VENTRICLE

EPENDYMAL

"DOWN" SPINAL CANAL

"UP" LEPTOMENINGES
ARACHNOID → SAS

ARACHNOID GRANULATIONS

DRAIN CSF

HYDROCEPHALUS

NPH = WACKY, WOBBLY, WET | VP SHUNT | LP DIAGNOSIS
- -
OBSTRUCTIVE → MASS | PROXIMA DILATE ONLY
COMMUNICATING ALL DILATE (SULCI DON'T)
→ ARACHNOID GRANULATIONS | (H/O MENINGITIS) SAH

HYDROCEPHALUS EX VACUO → ATROPHY | ALL DILATE EQUALLY

DURA + FALX

- CEREBRAL FALX
- L + R HEMISPHERES ABOVE CORPUS CALLOSUM
- TENTORIUM CEREBELLI CEREBELLUM + POSTERIOR LOBE
- TENTORIAL NOTCH – GAP IN WHICH BRAINSTEM IS IN

DURAL VENOUS SINUSES

SUPERIOR SAGITTAL SINUS AS EXAMPLE
VEINS FROM SCALP = EMISSARY
SKULL = DIPLOIC
MENINGES = MENINGEAL
CEREBRUM = BRIDGING

CSF VIA AG

DRAINAGE

SUPERIOR SAGITTAL	SUPERIOR CEREBRAL FALX	SKULL	CONFLUENCE
INFERIOR SAGITTAL	INFERIOR CEREBRAL FALX	CORPUS CALLOSUM	STRAIT
STRAIT	TENTORIUM CEREBELLI	N/A	CONFLUENCE

↑ INTO CONFLUENCE

↓ OUT OF CONFLUENCE

TRANSVERSE	OUTER TENTORIUM	SKULL	SIGMOID
SIGMOID		SKULL	INTERNAL JUGULAR

CAVERNOUS SINUS PATH

MENINGITIS →
PITUITARY
PARALYZED EYES — CAVERNOUS SINUS SYNDROME
↓ FACIAL SENSATION
+ HORNER'S
THROMBOSIS
DURAL VENOUS → ↑ ICP = HEADACHE PAPILLEDEMA

"" → EYES, NASAL CAVITY, ORBIT UPPER LIP ORAL MUCOSA
III EYE MOVEMENT + PNS
IV EYE MOVEMENT
V SENSORY FACE
VI EYE MOVEMENT

Intracranial Pressure, Cerebral Edema, and Brain Bleeds

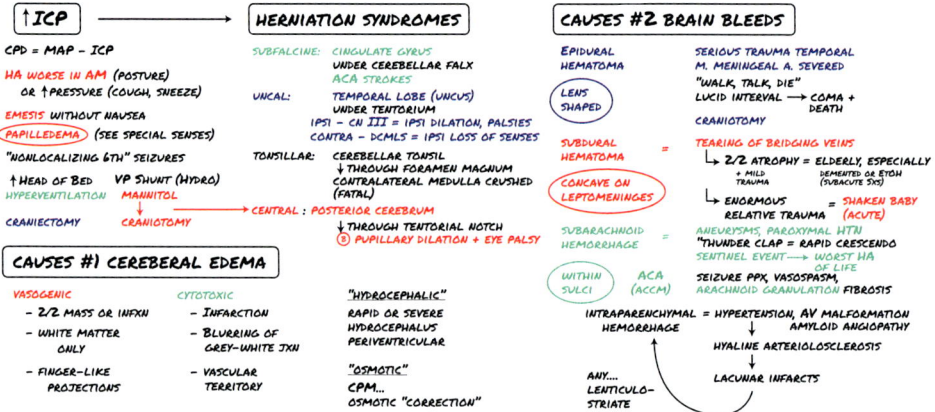

↑ ICP

CPD = MAP – ICP

HA WORSE IN AM (POSTURE) OR ↑PRESSURE (COUGH, SNEEZE)

EMESIS WITHOUT NAUSEA

PAPILLEDEMA (SEE SPECIAL SENSES)

"NONLOCALIZING 6TH" SEIZURES

↑HEAD OF BED | VP SHUNT (HYDRO)
HYPERVENTILATION | MANNITOL

CRANIECTOMY | CRANIOTOMY

CAUSES #1 CEREBERAL EDEMA

VASOGENIC
- 2/2 MASS OR INFXN
- WHITE MATTER ONLY
- FINGER–LIKE PROJECTIONS

CYTOTOXIC
- INFARCTION
- BLURRING OF GREY–WHITE JXN
- VASCULAR TERRITORY

HERNIATION SYNDROMES

SUBFALCINE: CINGULATE GYRUS UNDER CEREBELLAR FALX ACA STROKES

UNCAL: TEMPORAL LOBE (UNCUS) UNDER TENTORIUM
IPSI – CN III = IPSI DILATION, PALSIES
CONTRA – DCMLS = IPSI LOSS OF SENSES

TONSILLAR: CEREBELLAR TONSIL ↓ THROUGH FORAMEN MAGNUM CONTRALATERAL MEDULLA CRUSHED (FATAL)

CENTRAL: POSTERIOR CEREBRUM ↓ THROUGH TENTORIAL NOTCH ®PUPILLARY DILATION + EYE PALSY

"HYDROCEPHALIC" RAPID OR SEVERE HYDROCEPHALUS PERIVENTRICULAR

"OSMOTIC" CPM... OSMOTIC "CORRECTION"

CAUSES #2 BRAIN BLEEDS

EPIDURAL HEMATOMA
LENS SHAPED

SUBDURAL HEMATOMA =
CONCAVE ON LEPTOMENINGES

SUBARACHNOID HEMORRHAGE =
WITHIN SULCI | ACA (ACCM)

INTRAPARENCHYMAL = HYPERTENSION, AV MALFORMATION HEMORRHAGE

ANY.... LENTICULO-STRIATE

SERIOUS TRAUMA TEMPORAL M. MENINGEAL A. SEVERED
"WALK, TALK, DIE"
LUCID INTERVAL → COMA + DEATH
CRANIOTOMY

TEARING OF BRIDGING VEINS
↳ 2/2 ATROPHY = ELDERLY, ESPECIALLY + MILD TRAUMA | DEMENTED OR ETOH (SUBACUTE SXS)
↳ ENORMOUS RELATIVE TRAUMA = SHAKEN BABY (ACUTE)

ANEURYSMS, PAROXYMAL HTN
"THUNDER CLAP = RAPID CRESCENDO
SENTINEL EVENT → WORST HA OF LIFE
SEIZURE PPX, VASOSPASM,
ARACHNOID GRANULATION FIBROSIS

↓ AMYLOID ANGIOPATHY
HYALINE ARTERIOLOSCLEROSIS
↓
LACUNAR INFARCTS

NOTES

BASAL GANGLIA

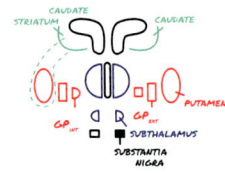

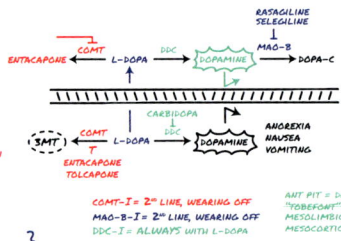

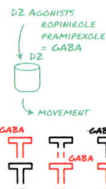

CAUDATE
STRIATUM   CAUDATE

PUTAMEN

GP INT   GP EXT
SUBTHALAMUS
SUBSTANTIA NIGRA

COMT
ENTACAPONE   L-DOPA   DDC   DOPAMINE   DOPA-C

RASAGILINE
SELEGILINE
MAO-B

D2 AGONISTS
ROPINIROLE
PRAMIPEXOLE
D2 = GABA

↓ MOVEMENT

3MT   COMT   L-DOPA   DDC   DOPAMINE   ANOREXIA
T   CARBIDOPA   NAUSEA
ENTACAPONE   VOMITING
TOLCAPONE

GABA   GABA

GABA   GABA
D2   D2   D2

COMT-I = 2ND LINE, WEARING OFF
MAO-B-I = 2ND LINE, WEARING OFF
DDC-I = ALWAYS WITH L-DOPA

ANT PIT = DOPAMINE-R = NO PROLACTIN
"FOBEFONT"
MESOLIMBIC: HALLUCINATIONS
MESOCORTICAL " C/₃ SXS

PARKINSON'S

PATH : α SYNUCLEIN AGGREGATES
SUBSTANTIA NIGRA 1ST
AGGREGATES = APOPTOSIS
NO DOPAMINE = NO GO

PT : PARKINSONISM = BRADYKINESIA
↳ SHUFFLING STEPS
↳ MASK-LIKE FACE
↳ PILL-ROLLING TREMOR
↳ COG WHEEL RIGIDITY
> 65 YO USUAL, COMMON
< 65 UNUSUAL, BUT NOT UNCOMMON

DX : CLINICAL
RADIO: MRI
BEST: BRAIN BIOPSY-
AUTOPSY

TX : PARKINSON'S DISEASE

NONE

TX : PARKINSONISM
> 65 LEVODOPA
CARBIDOPA
< 65 D2 AGONISTS

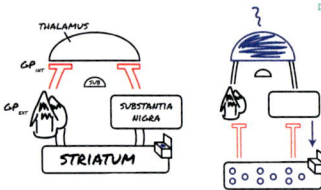

THALAMUS

GP INT

SUB

GP EXT   SUBSTANTIA NIGRA

STRIATUM

EPISODE 4: A NEW HOPE
(DIRECT PATH = MOVEMENT)

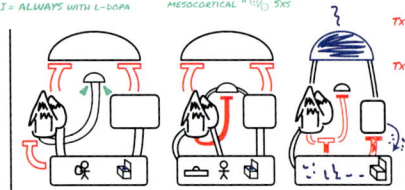

THALAMUS IS
DISINHIBITED
BY DOPAMINE (D2)

EPISODE 3: REVENGE OF THE DOPAMINE
(INDIRECT PATH = NO MOVEMENT)

Motor Systems

MOTOR CORTEX = FRONTAL LOBE

PRIMARY MOTOR CORTEX

↳ PRECENTRAL GYRUS
ANTERIOR TO CENTRAL SULCUS

↳ PYRAMIDAL NEURONS
(MULTIPOLAR)

↳ TORSO (WATERSHED)
HAND   LEG | FALX
FT | ACA
MCA   FACE

TEMPORAL

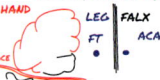

FRONTAL LOBE IN GENERAL

ATTENTION   THOUGHT
COGNITION   REASONING
INHIBITION   PERSONALITY
CONNECTS TO LIMBIC-REWARD EMOTION
BEHAVIOR
TO AMYGDALA MEMORY

CORTICOSPINAL TRACT

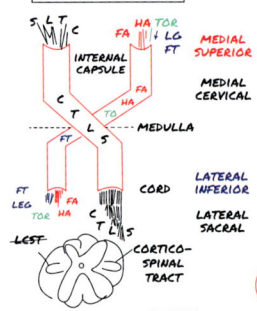

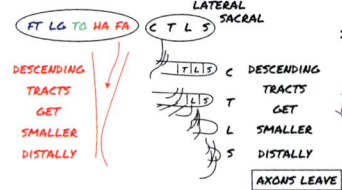

S L T C   HA TOR
FA ↓ LG
INTERNAL   FT
CAPSULE   MEDIAL
SUPERIOR
FA
C   HA   MEDIAL
T   TO   CERVICAL
L
FT   5   MEDULLA

FT   FA   CORD   LATERAL
LEG   TOR HA   INFERIOR
C T L 5

LEFT   LATERAL
SACRAL
CORTICO-
SPINAL
TRACT

LATERAL
SACRAL
FT LG TO HA FA   C T L 5

DESCENDING   T L 5 C
TRACTS   T
GET   L
SMALLER   5   DESCENDING
DISTALLY   TRACTS
GET
SMALLER
DISTALLY

AXONS LEAVE

CORD

CERVICAL – MOST WHITE MATTER
LARGEST SIZE

THORACIC –

LUMBAR – GREATEST GREY:WHITE

SACRAL – CONA MEDULLARIS
CAUDA EQUINA

MOTOR NEURON LESIONS IN CORD

– ABOVE LESION = NORMAL
– CONTRALATERAL = NORMAL
CORD

– AT THE LESION = LMN
IPSILATERAL
HYPOTONIC WEAKNESS
AREFLEXIA – ± ↑TOES

– BELOW THE LESION = UMN
IPSILATERAL
HYPERTONIC WEAKNESS
HYPERREFLEXIA
↑TOES

NOTES

Sensory Systems

SOMATO-SENSORY CORTEX + PARIETAL LOBE

PRIMARY SOMATOSENSORY CORTEX
→ POST-CENTRAL GYRUS
POSTERIOR TO CENTRAL SULCUS
+ "OTHER"

THALAMUS

STT
PAIN/TEMP

DCMLS
GENERALIZED TOUCH
VIBRATION
PROPRIOCEPTION

SENSE RECEPTORS

MECHANICAL
TACTILE = FINE TOUCH, VIB
MERKEL = TOUCH

PAIN
THERMAL   CHEMICAL

TEMP
COLD

STRONG
PRESSURE

(KRAUSE)

DEEP PRESSURE = LAMELLATED
VIBRATION = BULBOUS

"SENSORY CORTICOSPINAL"

DCMLS
FT T HA   T L S
C

NUCLEUS GRACILIS
CUNEATE NUCLEUS
CUNEATE FASCICLE

FASCICULUS GRACILIS

CORTICO
C C
T T
L L
S S

STT

ALWAYS CONTRA-LATERAL LOSS

NEURAL CREST

FT T HA FA

SLTC   CTLS
SLTC   CTLS

ASSESSING SENSATION

LESION ABOVE MEDULLA
↓ SENSATIONS CONGRUENT
CONTRALATERAL

LESION BELOW MEDULLA
↓ SENSATIONS INCONGRUENT
IPSI GENERAL   CONTRA PAIN/TEMP

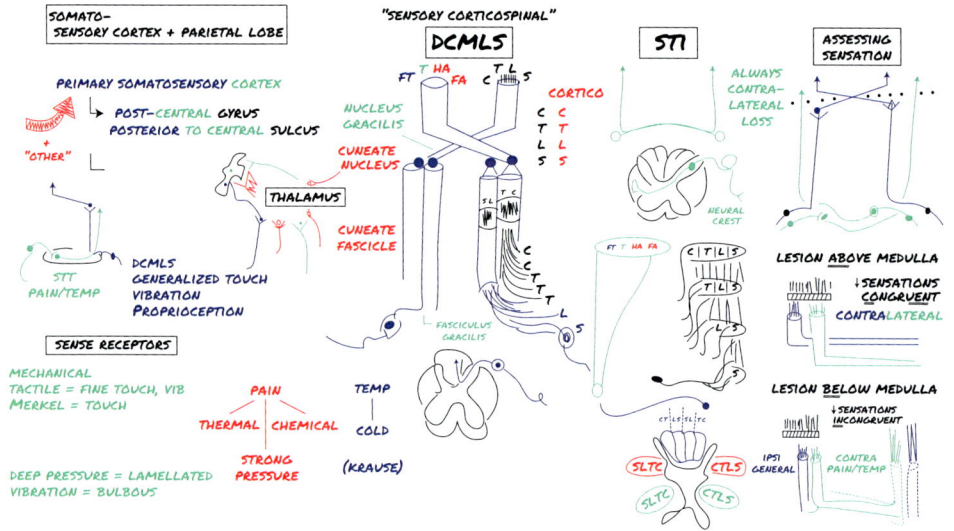

Spinal Cord Lesions

SPINE + SPINAL CORD
① VERTEBRAL BODIES CORTICAL + TRABECULAR PROTECTION
② INTERVERTEBRAL DISC NUCLEUS PULPOSUS (NOTOCHORD) *POTENTIAL HERNIATION
③ "MENINGES"
LEPTOMENINGES (CSF)
DURA MATER
VERTEBRAE (BONE)

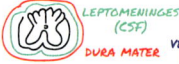

B_{12} DEFICIENCY + 3° SYPH
STT
22 YO ♀ VEGAN   55 YO "RAKE"
CST
IF NOT CORRECTED...CST
B_{12} DEFICIENCY   STT
(PERNICIOUS ANEMIA) ALSO DEMYELINATED

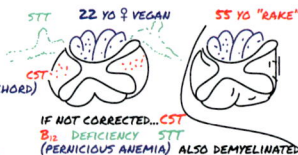

ALS
PATH : PROTEIN AGGREGATES
* NEURO - COGNITIVE - DEGENERATIVE DISORDER
1ST AFFECTED = α - MOTORNEURONS

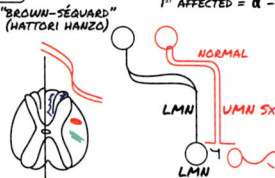

NORMAL
LMN   UMN Sx
LMN

NO TREATMENT
AGGREGATES INDUCE APOPTOSIS

DCMLS SPARED
ASA
AKA
⊗ STT
⊗ CORTICOSPINAL
ASA

RULES OF THE GAME
SPINAL CORD
→ CONTRALATERAL STT
→ IPSILATERAL DCMLS
→ @ LESION LMN
→ BELOW UMN
→ ABOVE NORMAL
= HEMISECTION
"BROWN-SÉQUARD" (HATTORI HANZO)

ADAMKIEWICZ (SP)
① RADICULAR
↳ NERVE ROOTS
② SEGMENTAL MEDULLARY
→ RADICULAR "PLUS" LUMBAR
→ ANTERIOR = ASA CISTERN
→ POSTERIOR = PSA (EITHER)
③ RADICULAR MEDULLARY

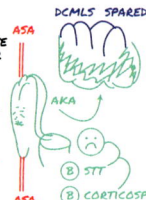

CAUDA EQUINA
L3   L3
CSF
DURA MATER
FILUM TERMINALE

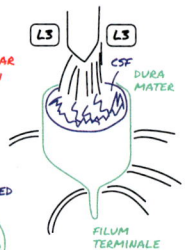

CAUDA EQUINA SYNDROME
PATH : COMPRESSION OF NERVES BY [ANYTHING]
PT : SADDLE ANESTHESIA
URINARY INCONTINENCE
[ANYTHING NEURAL]
"BACK PAIN"
DX : MRI
TX : SURGERY

Neuroscience

Cerebral Vasculature and Strokes

CIRCULATIONS + STROKES

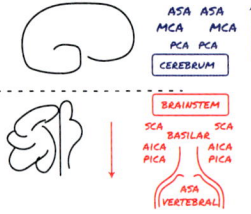

ASA   ASA
MCA   MCA
PCA   PCA
CEREBRUM

SCA   SCA
BASILAR
AICA   AICA
PICA   PICA

ASA
VERTEBRAL
BRAINSTEM

CIRCLE OF WILLIS

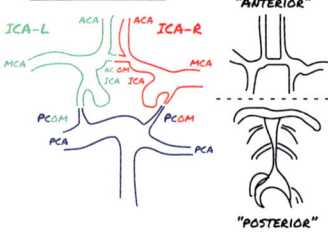

ICA-L   ACA   ACA   ICA-R
MCA   MCA
AC OM
ICA ICA
PCOM   PCOM
PCA   PCA

"ANTERIOR"

"POSTERIOR"

ACA

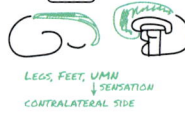

LEGS, FEET, UMN
↓ SENSATION
CONTRALATERAL SIDE

MCA

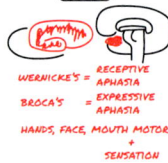

WERNICKE'S = RECEPTIVE APHASIA
BROCA'S = EXPRESSIVE APHASIA
HANDS, FACE, MOUTH MOTOR + SENSATION

PCA

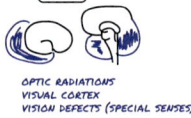

OPTIC RADIATIONS
VISUAL CORTEX
VISION DEFECTS (SPECIAL SENSES)

STROKE MECHANISMS   LACUNAR

HEMORRHAGIC = BLEED
- - - - - - - - - - - - - - - -

ISCHEMIC

→ EMBOLIC (AFIB, CAS)
  AFIB – ATRIAL APPENDAGE (CHA_2DS_2-VASC)
                                    (NOAC OR WARFARIN)
  CAS – ATHEROSCLEROSIS... RUPTURE, THROMBOSIS + EMBOLISM

→ THROMBOTIC = ATHEROSCLEROSIS

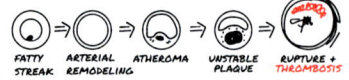

FATTY   ARTERIAL   ATHEROMA   UNSTABLE   RUPTURE +
STREAK   REMODELING   PLAQUE   THROMBOSIS

REVERSIBLE	IRREVERSIBLE	
HTN DM	AGE > 45 (M) > 55 (F)	ASA
TOBACCO	FAM HX	STATIN
OBESITY	GENES	RISK FACTOR
LIPIDS		MODIFICATION

TIA = RESOLUTION + NO EVIDENCE
      OF SXS ═══ MRI

→ LACUNAR = HYALINE ARTERIOLOSCLEROSIS

LENTICULOSTRIATE
GROSS = SMALL HOLES IN TISSUE
PREDISPOSES TO HEMORRHAGE

Cranial Nerves

CRANIAL NERVES

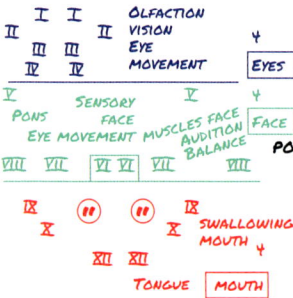

I   I   OLFACTION
II   II   VISION
III   III   EYE
IV   IV   MOVEMENT   EYES

V   V
PONS   SENSORY
        FACE
EYE MOVEMENT MUSCLES FACE
             AUDITION
             BALANCE   FACE

VIII VII   VI VI VII   VIII

IX   IX
X   X   SWALLOWING
                    MOUTH
XII   XII
         TONGUE   MOUTH

MOTOR: MEDIAL
SENSORY: LATERAL

ELEVEN DOESN'T COUNT
SIX IS OUT OF PLACE

CRANIAL FOSSAE

ANTERIOR CRIBRIFORM PLATE (I)
MIDDLE   OPTIC CHIASM (II)
          SUPERIOR ORBITAL
          FISSURE (III, IV, V_1)

          FORAMEN ROTUNDUM (V_2)
          FORAMEN OVALE (V_3)

POSTERIOR AUDITORY MEATUS (VII, VIII)
           JUGULAR FORAMEN
              (IX, X, XI)
           FORAMEN MAGNUM (XII)

CRANIAL NERVES

① PERIPHERAL NERVES
   OF THE CRANIUM
② SHARE THE BURDEN

MOTOR	SENSORY	MIXED
III	I	V
IV	II	VII
VI	VIII	IX
XII		X

TRIGEMINAL NERVE

SENSORY   FACE

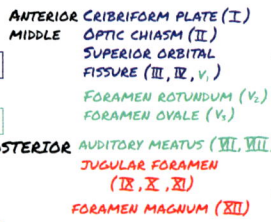

OPTHALMIC   MANDIBULAR
V_1 V_3

MAXILLARY
V_2

V_1 : FOREHEAD
     ORBIT, TOP OF NOSE

V_2 : EVERYTHING ELSE

V_3 MANDIBLE MOUTH, TONGUE
     LINGUAL NERVE (VII)

FACIAL NERVE

FACIAL: MOTOR FACE
          +
PARASYMPATHETIC
SALIVARY GLANDS
(NOT PAROTID)
          +
TASTE SENSATION
ANTERIOR 2/3 TONGUE
(CHORDAE TYMPANI)

CHORDAE TYMPANI

FACIAL SPLITS WITHIN
PAROTID, DOES NOT
INNERVATE

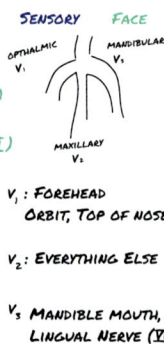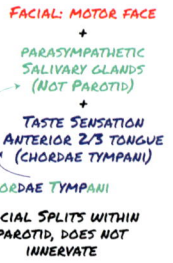

ANT
2/3

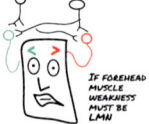

IF FOREHEAD
MUSCLE
WEAKNESS
MUST BE
LMN

→ SUPERIOR COLLICULI: (EYES)
→ INFERIOR COLLICULI: (EARS)

CEREBELLUM

PONS + CEREBELLUM

└→ 4TH VENTRICLE

MIDBRAIN

↳ CEREBRAL   ↳ PERIAQUEDUCTAL
  AQUEDUCT   GREY

↳ * CEREBRO-PONTO-
    CEREBELLAR TRACTS

↳ "TEGMENTUM"   ↳ "TECTUM"
  (FRONT)   (BACK)

↳ PONS = TRACTS
       ≠ BRIDGE

↳ BASIS PEDUNCULI   MOTOR
  CEREBRAL PEDUNCLES AXONS
  CRUS CEREBRI

⊘ CN V, VI, VII, VIII

METENCEPHALON

↳ SUBSTANTIA NIGRA

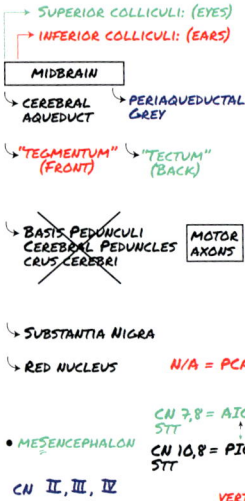

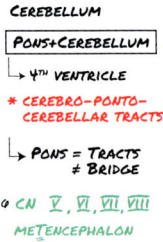

BRAINSTEM VASCULATURE

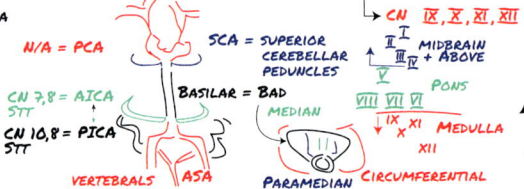

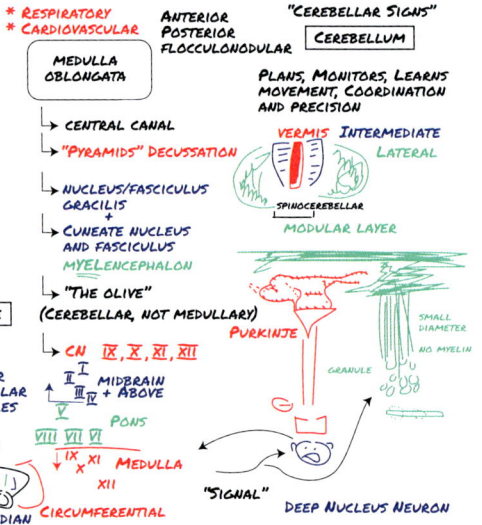

↳ RED NUCLEUS

N/A = PCA

SCA = SUPERIOR
      CEREBELLAR
      PEDUNCLES

• MESENCEPHALON

CN 7,8 = AICA
STT   BASILAR = BAD
CN 10,8 = PICA   MEDIAN
STT

CN II, III, IV

VERTEBRALS ASA

PARAMEDIAN CIRCUMFERENTIAL

* RESPIRATORY
* CARDIOVASCULAR

ANTERIOR
POSTERIOR
FLOCCULONODULAR

MEDULLA
OBLONGATA

↳ CENTRAL CANAL
↳ "PYRAMIDS" DECUSSATION

↳ NUCLEUS/FASCICULUS
  GRACILIS
  +
↳ CUNEATE NUCLEUS
  AND FASCICULUS
  MYELENCEPHALON

↳ "THE OLIVE"
  (CEREBELLAR, NOT MEDULLARY)

↳ CN IX, X, XI, XII

  II I
  III IV   MIDBRAIN
         + ABOVE
  V
  VIII VII VI   PONS
  IX XI   MEDULLA
  X
  XII

"CEREBELLAR SIGNS"

CEREBELLUM

PLANS, MONITORS, LEARNS
MOVEMENT, COORDINATION
AND PRECISION

VERMIS INTERMEDIATE
          LATERAL

SPINOCEREBELLAR

MODULAR LAYER

PURKINJE

GRANULE

SMALL
DIAMETER

NO MYELIN

"SIGNAL"   DEEP NUCLEUS NEURON

Brainstem Strokes

RULES OF BRAINSTEM

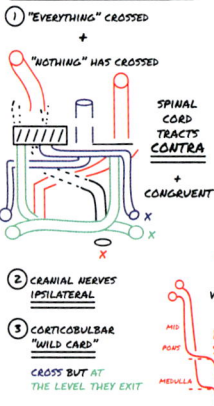

① "EVERYTHING" CROSSED
  +
  "NOTHING" HAS CROSSED

SPINAL
CORD
TRACTS
CONTRA
  +
CONGRUENT

② CRANIAL NERVES
  IPSILATERAL

③ CORTICOBULBAR
  "WILD CARD"

CROSS BUT AT
THE LEVEL THEY EXIT

MID
PONS
MEDULLA

MEDIAL MEDULLARY

"ASA" STROKE

ALL LIES... LEARN THE
"CLASSIC" ILLNESS SCRIPT

PT: UNILATERAL LOSS OF
    CONTRALATERAL CST
    CONTRALATERAL DCMLS
    SPARED STT
    HYPOGLOSSAL N. IPSI

LATERAL MEDULLARY

PICA

DESCENDING   IPSILATERAL
SYMPATHETIC   HORNER'S
INFERIOR   IPSILATERAL ATAXIA
CEREBELLAR   FALLS TO LESIONED SIDE
TRACTS
CORTICOBULBAR TT IPSILATERAL (FACE)
            STT CONTRALATERAL (BODY)
                 PAIN TEMP LOST
VESTIBULOCOCHLEAR IPSILATERAL VERTIGO
NUCLEUS   HEARING LOSS
DCMLS : SPARED
CST :   SPARED

DON'T
SOLVE   AWAY
*

NUCLEUS AMBIGUOUS
CN 9, 10

DYSARTHRIA, DYSPHAGIA
UVULA DEVIATION, AWAY

MEDIAL PONTINE

LOCKED IN SYNDROME

RETAINED : PAIN, SMELL, SIGHT
            COGNITION, EYELID LIFT
SPARED PAIN TEMP
BILATERAL LOSS CST
BILATERAL LOSS DCMLS
BILATERAL LOSS CORTICOBULBAR
            AND NUCLEI BELOW
            CN III

LATERAL PONTINE

AICA

SAME

SAME

SAME

SAME
(TOTAL DEAFNESS
IF LABRINTHINE)
SAME
SAME

NUCLEUS OF
FACIAL NERVE CN7

IPSILATERAL FACIAL DROOP
LOSS OF TASTE ANT 2/3 TONGUE

SUPERIOR CEREBELLAR A.

* CEREBELLAR SIGNS ONLY
  OVERSHOOT, DYSARTHRIA
  SPARED CST
  SPARED DCMLS
  SPARED STT

MEDIAL MIDBRAIN

SUPERIOR : EW NUCLEUS : IPSILATERAL
(WEBER)   LOSS PNS
                          = MYDRIASIS
        CN III : IPSILATERAL
                  "PALSY"
        DCMCS : CONTRALATERAL
                 HEMIPARESIS
CORTICOSPINAL : CONTRALATERAL
                 "HEMIPLEGIA"
        STT : SPARED

INFERIOR : EW : SAME
(BENEDICT) CN III : SAME
            DCMLS : SAME
CEREBELLAR TRACTS : HEMIATAXIA
                    MORE SO
                    THAN
                    HEMIPLEGIA
            STT : SAME

Intracranial Cancers

INTRACRANIAL CANCERS

- 1°
  - ADULTS = SUPRATENTORIAL
  - KIDS = INFRATENTORIAL
- METASTASIS TO BRAIN
  MOST COMMON

THE CANCER FORMERLY KNOWN...

GLIOBLASTOMA MULTIFORME (GBM)
PATH = EGFR → CDKN2A → TP53/RB
PT = SEIZURE/ FND → DEATH
                        1 YEAR
MRI = RING-ENHANCING
      CYSTIC/ NECROTIC
      CROSSES CORPUS
      SERPIGINOUS BORDER
HISTOLOGY = PSEUDOPALISADING
            PLEOMORPHIC NUCLEI
            AROUND NECROSIS
      "(+) GFAP"

ASTROCYTOMAS

"GRADE 1"	"GRADE 2"	"GRADE 3"	"GRADE 4"
LOCALIZED	HISTO DIFFUSE	ANAPLASTIC	GBM
CHILDREN	FOUND	ADULTS	ADULTS	ADULTS
EXCELLENT	PROGNO GOOD	POOR	< 1 YR

2° = GENE, GENE, GENE, GENE
                    1° = EGFR ↘
                           CDKN2A

OLIGODENDROGLIOMA

PATH : IDH 1/2 → TP53, RB
       WHITE MATTER
PT : SLOW, INDOLENT
     SEIZURE, FND
MRI : FRONTAL LOBE
      CALCIFICATION
HISTO : "FRIED EGG"
        ⊙

EPENDYMOMA

PATH :
PT : PEDIATRIC + OBSTRUCTIVE
     HYDROCEPHALUS
MRI : MASS IN 4TH VENTRICLE
HISTO : TRUE ROSETTES
        PERIVASCULAR PSEUDOROSETTES

MENINGIOMA

PATH : NF2, ♀:♂ 10:1
       NEURAL CREST (ARACHNOID)
PT : YOUNG ADULT ♀
     c̄ SEIZURE
MRI : WELL-CIRCUMSCRIBED
      NO PIA CONTACT
HISTO : NECROSIS
        WHORLS OF CELLS
        PSAMMOMA BODIES

MEDULLOBLASTOMA

PATH : WNT, β-CATENIN
       CEREBELLUM ONLY
PT : CEREBELLAR SIGNS
     ↑ICP, DROP METS
MRI : CEREBELLUM
      HYDROCEPHALUS
HISTO : GFAP, NEURONAL
        PEFFDN

PILOCYTIC ASTROCYTOMA

PATH : NOT EGFR/ TP53/ RB
       IS BRAF V600E
       SLOW-GROWING
PT : 4TH VENTRICLE = HYDROCEPHALUS
MRI : CEREBELLAR, HYDROCEPHALUS
HISTO : ROSENTHAL, WHO I
        "ACOUSTIC NEUROMA"

SCHWANNOMA

PATH : NF2, MERLIN
       ACOUSTIC MEATUS
PT : TINNITUS, DEAFNESS
MRI : Ⓑ SCHWANNOMA
HISTO : NON-MALIGNANT
        ANTONI A+B
        VEROCAY BODIES

CRANIOPHARYNGIOMA

PATH : RATHKE'S POUCH
       ANTERIOR PITUITARY
PT : BITEMPORAL
     HEMIANOPSIA
MRI : SELLA TURCICA
HISTO : CYSTIC + NON

GABA Receptors and Alcohol

GABA-R

GABA – A = Cl⁻
GABA – B = GPCR (G₅–cAMP)
GABA – C

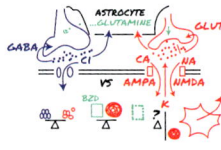

HYPERPOLARIZING

GABA-A + DRUGS

ONLY IN PRESENCE OF GABA
BZD = MORE FREQUENT
BARB = MORE DURATION

BENZO-BINDING DOMAINS

BZ 1 = CEREBRUM – SEDATIVE
       CEREBELLUM – ATAXIA
       HIPPOCAMPUS – ANTEROGRADE
       AMNESIA
BZ 2 = LIMBIC   ANXIOLYSIS
       ANTERIOR   MYORELAXANT
       HORN

GABA – GLUTAMANE BALANCE

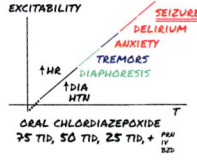

ASTROCYTE
...GLUTAMINE   GLUT
GABA
                   CA   NA
              VS AMPA NMDA
BZD

BENZO PHARM

MIDAZOLAM	FASTEST ACTING	MOST ADDICTING	PRE-OR
ALPRAZOLAM DIAZEPAM	FAST ON/OFF	PO TO ABORT/PREVENT PANIC ATTACKS
LORAZEPAM	MEDIUM ON/OFF	IV TO TX WITHDRAWAL P/M

SE: ANTEROGRADE AMNESIA
    RESPIRATORY DEPRESSION
ANTIDOTE: FLUMAZENIL * CAUSES SEIZURES

ZOLPIDEM SLEEP AIDS

WITHDRAWAL Sxs

EXCITABILITY   SEIZURE
                                DELIRIUM
                                ANXIETY
                                TREMORS
↑HR   DIAPHORESIS
  ↑DIA
  HTN
ORAL CHLORDIAZEPOXIDE
75 TID, 50 TID, 25 TID, + PRN IV BZD

BARBITURATES ARE BAD

THIOPENTAL INDUCTION
SHORT PROCEDURES

PHENOBARBITAL AS
2ND/3RD AED

LOW SAFETY
LOW UTILITY

ETOH

"DIRTY BENZO"
ATAXIA   ANXIOLYSIS
AMNESIA   MUSCLE
            RELAXATION
"HANGOVER" 2/2
METABOLITES (ALDEHYDE)
  CEREBELLAR VERMIS
  ATROPHY
  CEREBRAL ATROPHY
  ACCELERATED DEMENTIA
  B₁ DEFICIENCY =
  WERNICKE – KORSAKOFF
  (REVERSIBLE) (IRREVERSIBLE)

OTHER ALCOHOL

– METHANOL   MOONSHINE
  + AG MET ACID FORMATE
                 BLINDNESS
– ETHYLENE   ANTI-FREEZE
  GLYCOL   CA OXALATE STONES
+ AG MET   OBSTRUCTIVE
  ACID   NEPHROPATHY
                 WOOD'S LAMP
                 FOMEPIZOLE (ETOH)
– ISOPROPYL   CLEANING SOLVENT
  ALCOHOL   KETONEMIA/URIA
                 c̄ AG MET ACID

NOTES

SEIZURE

SYNCHRONIZATION OF
NEURAL TRACTS
(SAH)

VASCULAR — BLEED, STROKE, VASCULITIS
INFXN — MENINGITIS, ENCEPHALITIS
TRAUMA — TBI, CONCUSSION
AUTOIMMUNE — "SEROSITIS"
METABOLIC — ↓O_2, ↓GLUCOSE, NA, CA, OSM
INGESTION/WITHDRAWAL — ETOH BZD
NEOPLASM — * MENINGIOMA, ANY
PSYCH — PSEUDOSEIZURE

EPILEPSY

2+ SEIZURES WITHOUT
A SECONDARY CAUSE

DX: EEG   TRIGGERS:
↳ FOCAL   – LACK OF SLEEP
↳ FOCAL TO   – EMOTIONAL DISTRESS
  GENERAL   – STIMULANTS
↳ GENERALIZED   – FLASHES OF
                   LIGHT
TX: AEDS   – MENSES

"PARTIAL" ONSET

– FOCAL
  · UNILATERAL
    HEMISPHERE
  · ANY TRACT
– FOCAL TO
  GENERALIZED
  · UNILATERAL
    HEMISPHERE
  · GRADUALLY
    PROGRESSES
  JACKSONIAN MARCH
  SECONDARILY GENERALIZED
  – GENERALIZED
    BILATERAL
    HEMISPHERES

AWARENESS

RETAINED
AWARENESS
(RECALLS EVENTS)
"SIMPLE"

IMPAIRED
AWARENESS
(UNABLE RECALL)
"COMPLEX"

STATUS EPILEPTICUS

LIFE-THREATENING EMERGENCY
SEIZURE ACTIVITY CONTINUES
  FOR ≥5MIN 30MINS
  OR
TWO SEIZURES ? RETURN
  TO BASELINE
IF IMPROVING... LET THEM

*FOCAL ≡ ANYTHING

MOTOR

– MYOCLONIC
  <0.1 SECONDS
  MUSCLE JERK
– ATONIC
  "DROP SEIZURE"
  LOSS OF TONE
  PEDIATRIC
– TONIC
  SUSTAINED CONTRACTION
  >10 SECONDS
  FLEXION/EXTENSION
  OF ANY OR ALL
– CLONIC
  RHYTHMIC CONTRACTION
  2–5 SECOND INTERVALS
  "CONCLUSIONS"
– TONIC-CLONIC
  COMBINATION
  INCLUDES
  NEITHER
– NON MOTOR
  NO Δ IN TONE

"GRAND MAL"

GENERALIZED TONIC-CLONIC

GENERALIZED (IMPAIRED)
TONIC – CLONIC – REST
SOME: AURA
ALL: POST ICTAL STATE

TONGUE — INCONTINENCE — LIMB
BITING — JERKING
          "ABSENCE"

GENERALIZED NON-MOTOR

GENERALIZED (IMPAIRED)
NONMOTOR   RETAINED
  OR   +   TONE
AUTOMATISMS
          +
       BLANK STARE
5–15 SECONDS, 100/DAY

ADHD   SEIZURES
       ETHOSUXIMIDE

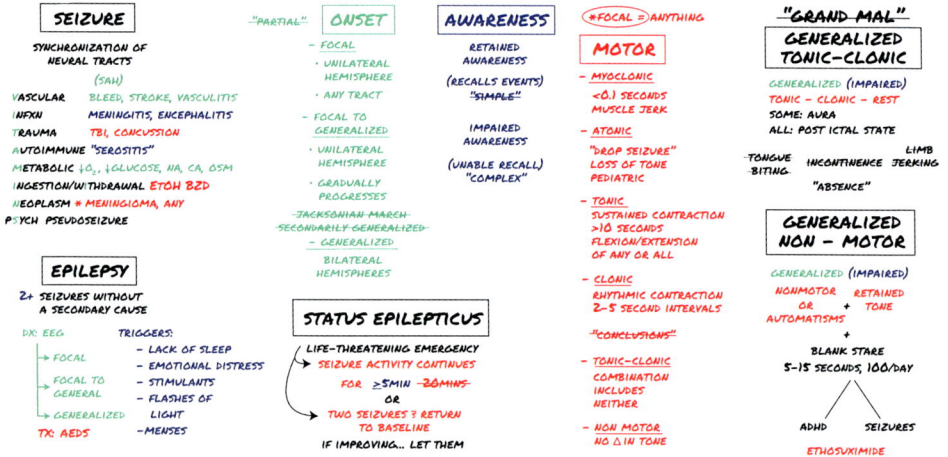

Seizure Pharmacology

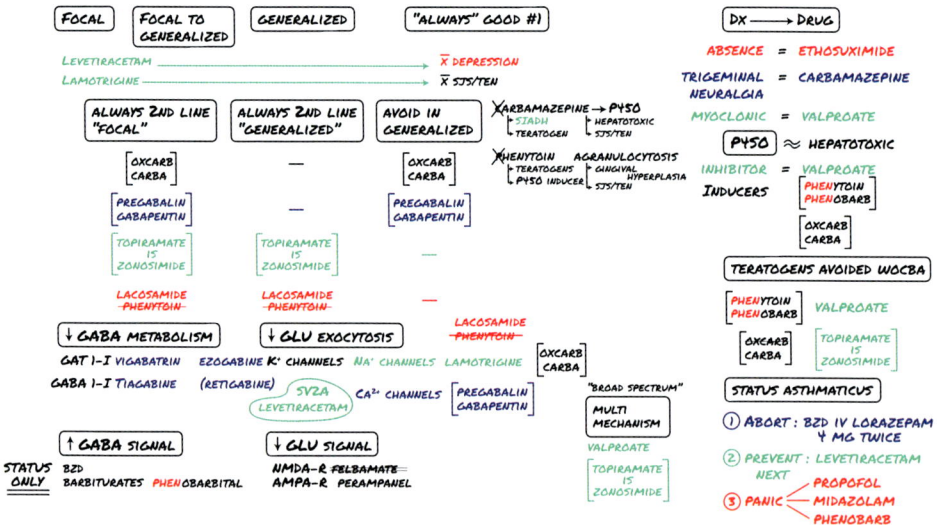

FOCAL	FOCAL TO GENERALIZED	GENERALIZED	"ALWAYS" GOOD #1		DX ⟶ DRUG

LEVETIRACETAM ———————————————→ X̄ DEPRESSION
LAMOTRIGINE ———————————————→ X̄ SJS/TEN

ALWAYS 2ND LINE "FOCAL"	ALWAYS 2ND LINE "GENERALIZED"	AVOID IN GENERALIZED
OXCARB CARBA	—	OXCARB CARBA
PREGABALIN GABAPENTIN	—	PREGABALIN GABAPENTIN
TOPIRAMATE IS ZONOSIMIDE	TOPIRAMATE IS ZONOSIMIDE	—
LACOSAMIDE PHENYTOIN	LACOSAMIDE PHENYTOIN	—

CARBAMAZEPINE → P450
  ⌐ SIADH   ⌐ HEPATOTOXIC
  L TERATOGEN   L SJS/TEN

PHENYTOIN   AGRANULOCYTOSIS
  ⌐ TERATOGENS   ⌐ GINGIVAL HYPERPLASIA
  L P450 INDUCER L SJS/TEN
                          LACOSAMIDE
                          PHENYTOIN

↓ GABA METABOLISM
GAT 1–I VIGABATRIN
GABA 1–I TIAGABINE

↑ GABA SIGNAL
STATUS   BZD
ONLY   BARBITURATES PHENOBARBITAL

↓ GLU EXOCYTOSIS
EZOGABINE K⁺ CHANNELS   Na⁺ CHANNELS LAMOTRIGINE
(RETIGABINE)   OXCARB
         SV2A   CA²⁺ CHANNELS CARBA
  LEVETIRACETAM   PREGABALIN
                        GABAPENTIN

↓ GLU SIGNAL
NMDA–R FELBAMATE
AMPA–R PERAMPANEL

"BROAD SPECTRUM"
MULTI MECHANISM
VALPROATE
TOPIRAMATE
IS
ZONOSIMIDE

ABSENCE = ETHOSUXIMIDE
TRIGEMINAL = CARBAMAZEPINE
NEURALGIA
MYOCLONIC = VALPROATE

P450 ≈ HEPATOTOXIC

INHIBITOR = VALPROATE
INDUCERS   PHENYTOIN PHENOBARB
           OXCARB CARBA

TERATOGENS AVOIDED WOCBA

PHENYTOIN PHENOBARB   VALPROATE
OXCARB CARBA   TOPIRAMATE IS ZONOSIMIDE

STATUS ASTHMATICUS

1 ABORT : BZD IV LORAZEPAM
          4 MG TWICE
2 PREVENT : LEVETIRACETAM
  NEXT   ⌐ PROPOFOL
3 PANIC ⟨ MIDAZOLAM
                    L PHENOBARB

N O T E S

Headache

HA → RED FLAGS

Ø → 1° HEADACHE

⊕ → FEVER / FND / PAPILLEDEMA → 2° HEADACHE — IMAGING

1° HEADACHE

CLUSTER
- MECH: ?? M>F, NOT TRIGEMINAL
- PT: UNILATERAL EXTREME PAIN SUPRAORBITAL + IPSILATERAL AUTONOMIC DYSFXN
- DUR: 15 MINS – 3 HRS
- ATTACK: 6–10 / DAY
- ACUTE TX: 100% O₂, TRIPTANS
- PPX: VERAPAMIL

MIGRAINE
- MECH: ?? "AURAS" "POST-ICTAL" "TRIGGERS"
- PT: UNILATERAL THROBBING PAIN... ± AURA
  - ⊕ PHOTOPHOBIA
  - ⊕ PHONOPHOBIA
  - N/V
- DUR: 4 – 72 HRS
- TRIGGERS, LACK OF SLEEP STIMULANTS
- NSAIDS / ACETAMINOPHEN
  - *CAD
  - TRIPTANS
  - ERGOTAMINE
- PPX: PROPANOLOL, AVOID TRIGGERS, VALPROATE, TOPIRAMATE, VENLAFAXINE

TENSION
- PT: BILATERAL FOREHEAD BAND
- RARELY SEEN B/C TAKES CARE OF ITSELF
- DUR: 4–6 HRS

TRIGEMINAL NEURALGIA
- MECH: ??
- PT: ELECTRIC SHOCKS FACE PAIN DISTRIBUTION OF V₁ V₂ V₃ PROVOKED CHEWING, TALKING, GENTLE TOUCH
- DUR: < 1 MIN
- ATTK: ↑FREQUENCY + INTENSITY
- ACUTE TX: _____
- PPX: CARBAMAZEPINE

2° HEADACHE — IMAGING
- FEVER + HA — CT LP BX
  - STIFF NECK MENINGITIS
  - AMS ENCEPHALITIS
  - FND ABSCESS
- FND + HA — CT MRI, BX
  - BLEED (ACUTE)
  - CANCER (CHRONIC)
- PAPILLEDEMA → ↑ICP, HA CT, MRI, BX

GIANT CELL ARTERITIS	IDIOPATHIC INTRACRANIAL HTN
AGE > 50 + IPSILATERAL JAW CLAUDICATION + PALPABLE NODULES	YOUNG (20–40) OBESE ♀
GIVE STEROIDS BX	DX CT ⊖
	LP = ↑PRESSURE
	TX: ACETAZOLAMIDE

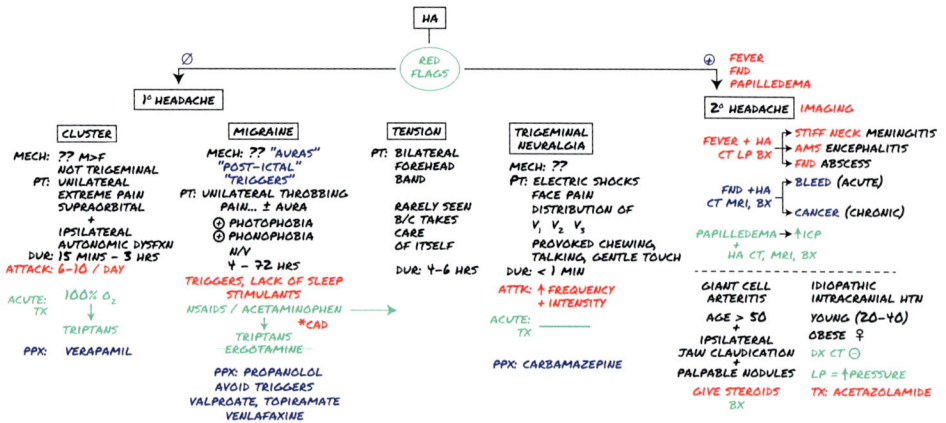

Neurocognitive Degeneration

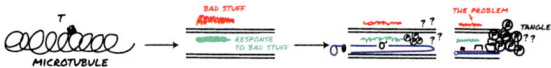

MICROTUBULE → BAD STUFF / RESPONSE TO BAD STUFF → ?? → THE PROBLEM / TANGLES ??

*ALS α-MOTOR NEURONS FIRST SOD TDP-43

ALZHEIMER'S
- PATH: Aβ PLAQUES (AGGREGATES) TAU TANGLES (SYMPTOMS) TEMPORAL LOBE (MEMORY)
  - SECRETIN α → γ = NORMAL
  - β → γ = Aβ
  - E₄ TRISOMY 21 = APP X 3
  - E₃ APO₄ : E₄E₄ BAD E₂E₂ GOOD
  - E₂
- PT: MEMORY + ATTENTION LOST FIRST – SHORT TERM MEMORY, ATTENTION. THEN – PROGRESSIVE RETROGRADE AMNESIA SOCIAL GRACES RETAINED
- DX: CT/ MRI ATROPHY *HIPPOCAMPUS + TEMPORAL LOBE. BEST = AUTOPSY PLAQUES + TANGLES
- TX: SYMPTOMS ONLY DONEPEZIL, MAMONTINE (ACHE-I) (GLUT AGONIST)

FTLDs
- PATH: TDP?? TAU?? TAU TANGLES FRONTAL LOBE (INHIBITION) LEAST WELL CHARACTERIZED SYNDROME "FTLD" NOT PATHOGENESIS
- PT: DISINHIBITION (ANTERIOR FRONTAL) + PERSONALITY Δ. LATE: ABSENT SPEECH (BROCA'S) ABSENT MOVEMENT (PMC). ALSO: MEMORY LOSS SOCIAL GRACES LOST
- DX: CT/MRI ATROPHY *FRONTAL LOBES. BEST = AUTOPSY PICK BODIES IN PICK CELLS
- TX: NONE

LEWY BODY DEMENTIA
- PATH: α-SYNUCLEIN AGGREGATES TAU TANGLES SUBSTANTIA NIGRA α-SYNUCLEIN (SNCA) PARKIN (PRKN)
  - LEWY BODY = DEMENTIA + PARKINSONISM
  - PARKINSON = PARKINSONISM + DEMENTIA
- PT: BRADYKINESIA PARKINSONISM
  - MASK-LIKE FACE
  - SHUFFLING STEPS
  - COG WHEEL RIGIDITY
  - PILL-ROLLING TREMOR
  - DEMENTIA PREDOMINATES
- DX: MRI ATROPHY SUBSTANTIA NIGRA. BEST = AUTOPSY
  - LEWY BODIES
  - TAU TANGLES
- TX: SXS ONLY PARKINSONISM

HUNTINGTON
- PATH: HUNTINGTIN AGGREGATES CAUDATE CHROMOSOME 4 HTT TRINUCLEOTIDE REPEAT EXPANSION (CAG) ANTICIPATION (SPERMATOGENESIS) AUTOSOMAL DOMINANT MORE CAG = EARLIER ONSET
- PT: HYPERKINESIA CHOREIFORM, BALLISTIC WRITHING OF ALL MUSCLES
- DX: GENETIC FIND CAG REPEATS. BEST: AUTOPSY → HUNTINGTIN AGGREGATES
- TX: NONE

168 © 2021 OnlineMedEd

Neuroscience

Pain and Analgesic Tracts

PAIN FIBERS

FAST FIBER : Aδ = CORTICAL SENSORY
- FREE NERVE ENDING
- LARGE + MYELINATED
- GLUTAMATE
- MAINLY TO THALAMUS THEN CORTEX
- SHARP, MAXIMAL INTENSITY, SHORT LIVED

SLOW FIBER : C = BULBAR SENSORY
- FREE NERVE ENDING
- SMALL RADIUS
- NO MYELIN
- ACT THROUGH SUBSTANCE P (MUST ACCUMULATE)
- MULTIPLE INTERNEURONS
- MAINLY TO BRAINSTEM TECTAL PERIAQUEDUCTAL GREY RETICULAR FORMATION
- SOME TO THALAMUS THEN CORTEX
- SUFFERING TRACT

ANALGESIA TRACT

"MOTOR" FOR PAIN "SENSORY"
PERI-VENTRICULAR NUCLEUS (HYPOTHALAMIC)

DOPAMINE ENKEPHALIN-RELEASING INTERNEURON (TEGMENTUM PERIAQUADUCTAL)

ENKEPHALIN RAPHE NUCLEUS, RETICULAR (PONS) FORMATION (PONS)

SEROTONIN ENKEPHALIN-RELEASING INTERNEURON (CORD)

ENKEPHALIN
SLOW PAIN FIBER (PRESYNAPTIC) → FAST + SLOW (POSTSYNAPTIC)

OPIATE INTOXICATION

NO UPPER LIMIT OF DOSE

μ1 = NO PAIN
μ2 = FEEL GOOD

NALOXONE REVERSAL

- CONSTRICTED "PINPOINT" PUPILS
- RESPIRATORY DEPRESSION → FEW, SHALLOW, CYANOSIS BREATHS —FATAL

MOR PHYSIOLOGY

PRESYNAPTIC ↑EXCITATORY NTS
MOR CLOSES CA BY ↓CAMP Gi

POSTSYNAPTIC HYPERPOLARIZATION
MOR OPENS K⁺ BY ↓CAMP Gi2

MOR
✓ μ1 = ACUTE PAIN, PALLIATION
  ↓ANALGESIA
  ↓DYSPNEA, ↓FEAR OF DYING
  μ2 = EUPHORIA DEPENDENCE TOLERANCE
  CONSTIPATION, MIOSIS, PRURITIS
  RESPIRATORY DEPRESSION
  μ3 = VASODILATION

DOR ENKEPHALIN SPINAL ANALGESIA
KOR DYNORPHIN DYSPHORIA

NOR NOCICEPTIN
HYPERALGESIA
UNLIKELY RELATED BY
SIMILAR PHYSIOLOGY

OPIATE WITHDRAWAL
PAIN, DYSPHORIA SUFFERING
N/V/D
NOT FATAL/NO SEIZURES

OPIATES
MORPHINE, CODEINE } WITHIN POPPY

OPIOIDS
FENTANYL → TD
HYDROMORPHONE → ORAL, LOLLIPOPS

II
MORPHINE
OXYCODONE
HYDROCODONE

CODEINE → COUGH
DEXTROMETHORPHAN

LOPERAMIDE - DIARRHEA TREATMENT

OPIOID TREATMENT
NALOXONE IMMEDIATE REVERSAL SHORT HALF-LIFE
NALTREXONE LONGER ACTING ORAL HIGHER AFFINITY MOR ↑ ACTIVATION
BUPRENORPHINE PARTIAL μ AGONIST, K ANTAGONIST
SUBOXONE NALTREXONE + BUPRENORPHINE
METHADONE REPLACEMENT THERAPY

Anesthesia

LOCAL ANESTHESIA
PREVENT TRANSMISSION OF PAIN TO SPINAL CORD
↳ BIND OPEN-INACTIVATED CHANNELS ↓ RETURN TO RESTING (1000x)
↳ ACT FROM WITHIN CYTOPLASM
↳ RESERVOIR CONCEPT. ARE WEAK BASES SO CAN PROTONATE AND DEPROTONATE TO CROSS AQUEOUS AND LIPID COMPARTMENTS *WORK WORSE IN ACIDIC
↳ USE-DEPENDENT (FREQUENCY) MORE EFFECTIVE ON MYELINATED (OF SAME SIZE) CONDUCTION VELOCITY MATTERS MOST
↳ SYSTEMIC TOXICITY = SEIZURE, METALLIC TASTE
+ EPINEPHRINE *WASHOUT (NOT OR DIGITS)

AMIDES : TOPICAL
COCAINE ARE
PROCAINE CONSTRICTORS
BENZOCAINE

LOCAL SUBQ MOST MINOR PROCEDURES

NERVE BLOCK: PUDENDAL

ESTERS : INJECTION OR INFUSION
+ LIDOCAINE BUPIVICAINE

EPIDURAL :
INFUSION, OR ⊕CSS

SPINAL ⊕CSC

INDUCTION
GABA_A   MOR
AMNESIA   ANALGESIA

PROPOFOL   FENTANYL
↳ SWINGS OF BP
↳ PRIS = "MITOCHONDRIA" ONLY WITH PROLONGED + HIGH DOSES
ETOMIDATE
↳ LIMITED Δ IN BP
↳ RSI
‾THIOPENTAL‾
?
- - - - - - - - - - - - -
CONSCIOUS SEDATION
OR
INDUCTION AUGMENTATION
IV MIDAZOLAM
KETAMINE FOR KIDS

INTUBATION
SK. MUSCLE   AUTONOMICS
PARALYTICS INHIBIT NACH-R

DEPOLARIZING
SUCCINYLCHOLINE
K⁺, RAPID ON
RAPID OFF
FASCICULATIONS

NON DEPOLARIZING
—CURONIUM
VEC NO K⁺
ROC CONCERNS
EMG MONITOR

MALIGNANT HYPERTHERMIA
NO GAS
DANTROLENE
RYANODINE OPEN
ALL MUSCLES
BUT ⊕ GENE?
NO GAS
TETANY
RHABDO, RENAL FAILURE
↑TEMP

MAINTENANCE
GAS
ISO — FLURANE
SEVO
- - - - - -
NITROUS OXIDE
HALOTHANE

- BLOOD-GAS PARTITION (SOLUBILITY) COEFFICIENT
↓SOLUBILITY (↑BGPC) = FASTER ONSET IN BLOOD

- OIL-GAS PARTITION (SOLUBILITY) COEFFICIENT
↑SOLUBILITY (↑BGPC) = ↑POTENCY IN BRAIN (NEEDLESS)

- MAC = 1 / OGPC → THANKS, MATH

- DEW = 1 / MAC → THIS IS A JOKE

© 2021 OnlineMedEd

The Eye—Anterior Eye

Anterior Anatomy

CORNEA — GLOBE
SCLERA — PUPIL
IRIS
LENS — * LIGHT
CILIARY BODY — REFRACTION

AQUEOUS HUMOR
—ANTERIOR CHAMBER
—POSTERIOR CHAMBER

VITREOUS HUMOR
INTRINSIC MUSCLES
  —IRIS DILATOR
  —IRIS SPHINCTER (SPHINCTER PUPILLAE)
  —CILIARY MUSCLE

Posterior Anatomy
RETINA (NEXT LESSON)
+ ALL THE THINGS

EXTRAOCULAR
  MUSCLES

Iris Controls Exposure
IRIS = STROMA ONLY ANTERIOR
  MELANOCYTES W/I STROMA
  "DOUBLE EPITHELIUM" PIGMENT
  POSTERIOR
  + MUSCLES IN BETWEEN

IRIS DILATOR M(M).... "DILATES PUPIL"

↑ APERTURE (SNS)

IRIS SPHINCTER M .... "CONSTRICTS PUPIL"

↑ APERTURE (PNS)

ENOUGH LIGHT TO ACTIVATE
PHOTORECEPTORS....
BUT NOT SO MUCH THE LIGHT
SEARS THEM

LOTS OF LIGHT... RELAXATION DILATORS
  CONTRACTION SPHINCTER

LITTLE LIGHT... CONTRACTION DILATORS
  RELAXATION SPHINCTER

Lens Controls Focus
PIGMENTED HOLDS ZONULE
EPITHELIUM FIBERS

CILIARY = SPHINCTER
MUSCLE

CONTRACTION = CLOSES APERTURE
  LOOSENING TENSION
  SPHERICAL LENS

RELAXATION = OPENS APERTURE
  STRETCHING FIBERS
  FLATTENING LENS

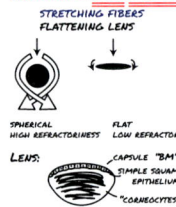

SPHERICAL — FLAT
HIGH REFRACTORINESS — LOW REFRACTORINESS

LENS: CAPSULE "BM"
  SIMPLE SQUAMOUS
  EPITHELIUM
  "CORNEOCYTES"

Aqueous Humor
BATHES INNER CORNEA
CORNEA
  TRABECULAR MESHWORK
  CANAL OF SCHLEMM

LENS
BATHES
LENS

99% WATER
(NO Δ VISION)
GLUCOSE, IONS,
VITAMINS

EPENDYMAL OF THE CHOROID MAKE CSF
  CELLS — PLEXUT — AQUEOUS
  NONPIGMENTED — CILIARY — HUMOR
  EPITHELIAL — PROCESSES
  CELLS

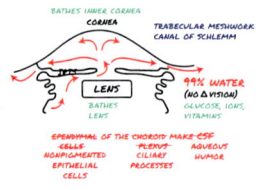

Conjunctiva + Eyelid
CORNEA EPITHELIUM		STRATIFIED SQUAMOUS, NO BASAL LAYER (MELANOCYTES), CORNEOCYTES
CONJUNCTIVAL EPITHELIUM		STRATIFIED SQUAMOUS + BASAL LAYER + PIGMENT, NO CORNEOCYTES
EYELID (SKIN) EPITHELIUM		KERATINIZED STRATIFIED SQUAMOUS + ALL

TEARS
LACRIMAL GLAND
LACRIMAL DUCT
+ TARSAL GLANDS (OILY) + ACCESSORY LACRIMAL GLANDS (WATER)

The Eye—Retina

Retina Layers
INNER LIMITING MEMBRANE
OUTPUT AXONS
GANGLION CELL LAYER
INNER PLEXIFORM LAYER
BIPOLAR CELL LAYER
OUTER PLEXIFORM LAYER
OUTER NUCLEAR LAYER
OUTER LIMITING MEMBRANE
RODS + CONES LAYER
LAYER OF PIGMENTED
  EPITHELIUM

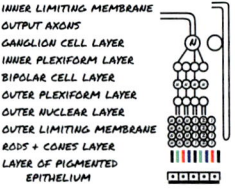

SIGNAL CONVERGENCE

Which We Care About
PHOTORECEPTOR ELEMENTS +
BIPOLAR NEURONS — NUCLEI
GANGLION NEURONS + GANGLION AXONS

HORIZONTAL
PIGMENTED EPITHELIUM
  ABSORBS EXCESS LIGHT
  PHAGOCYTOSIS PR ELEMENTS
  FEEDS RODS + CONES

Photoreceptors
—CONES
  RED CONES
  GREEN CONES — MITO-CHONDRIA
  BLUE CONES
  CILIA
CENTRAL
HIGH-ACUITY
CONE
—RODS
  LIGHT OR NOT
  PERIPHERAL
  LOW-ACUITY
ROD

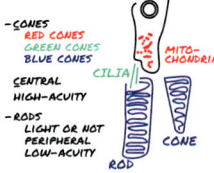

Acuity + Receptive Fields
RODS ONLY
FOVEA, CONES ONLY

NEEDS 5 — NEEDS 5
LOW-LIGHT — HIGH-LIGHT
LOW-ACUITY — HIGH-ACUITY

SAME
TOTAL
ΔING
%

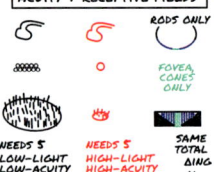

Photoreception
IN THE DARK = DEPOLARIZED
RETINAL INTACT
TRANSDUCIN OFF
PHOSPHODIESTERASE OFF
[cGMP] KEEPS NA+ CHANNELS OPEN

IN THE LIGHT = HYPERPOLARIZED
RETINAL → RHODOPSIN
TRANSDUCIN ON (GCPR Gₜ)
PHOSPHODIESTERASE ON

↓ [cGMP] CLOSES NA+ CHANNELS

Track + Field
(NOT TRUE!)
NO
TOUCHIE!

Ⓛ Ⓡ
FIELD FIELD

BLACK IS LOSS
OK

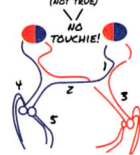

Extraocular MM.
RECTI
SUPERIOR RECTUS ↑
INFERIOR RECTUS ↓
MEDIAL RECTUS — MEDIALLY
LATERAL RECTUS — (ABDUCENS) LATERALLY

OBLIQUE:
INFERIOR OBLIQUE: UP AND OUT
SUPERIOR OBLIQUE: (TROCHLEA) DOWN AND OUT

PALSIES
TROCHLEAR N. PALSY
  UP + IN — TROUBLE LOOKING
  WITH A HEAD — DOWN
  TILT

ABDUCENS N. PALSY
  MEDIAL → FAILS TO CROSS
  ROTATION — MIDLINE

OCULOMOTOR N. PALSY
  NORMAL DOWN
  PUPIL + + BLOWN PUPIL
  (STROKE) OUT (COMPRESSION)

NOTES

The Eye—Eye Pathologies

OnlineMedEd

RED EYE

If RED FLAGS, REFER OUT
PAINFUL, BLURRY, PHOTOPHOBIA

① CONJUNCTIVITIS = CONJUNCTIVAL INJECTION

	DISCHARGE	ITCH	LATERALITY
VIRAL	WATERY	—	UNILATERAL
BACTERIAL	PURULENT	—	UNILATERAL
ALLERGIC	WATERY OR NONE	⊕	⊕

② SCLERITIS (SCLERAL INJECTION)
RED EYE + PAIN, Ø LIMBIC SPARING
PAIN ON MOVEMENT, Ø BLURRY/Ø PHOTO

③ EPISCLERITIS
FOCAL, PAINFUL, NOT LIFE-THREATENING
NSAIDS + GTTS

④ IRITIS (ANTERIOR UVEITIS) (CILIARY INJECTION)
RED EYE + PAIN, Ø LIMBIC SPARING
PAIN ON MOVEMENT ⊕ BLURRY/⊕ PHOTO

⑤ KERATITIS ("CORNEA-ITIS")
CONTACT LENS = PSEUDOMONAS INFXN
PUS IN ANTERIOR CHAMBER
CORNEAL ABRASION FLUORESCEIN DYE

CATARACT

PATH : MULTIPLE = DM, STEROIDS
SMOKING, AGE
CONGENITAL = METABOLIC

PT : PAINLESS BLURRED
VISION
OPACIFICATION OF LENS

DX : CLINICAL

TX : SURGERY

FOCUS

MYOPIA = NEAR-SIGHTED
TOO ROUND/EYE SHORT
TX ⊖ = POWER, CONVEX LENS

HYPEROPIA = FAR-SIGHTED
TOO FLAT/EYE LONG
TX ⊖ ⊕ POWER, CONCAVE LENS

ASTIGMATISM = CORNEA WARPED
REQUIRES SPECIFIC LENS
UNIQUE TO THAT CORNEA

PRESBIOPIA = OLD AGE
STIFF LENS, SEEING CLOSE
IS HARD

ACUTE ∡ GLAUCOMA

ALREADY ACUTE ∡
(NO ↑ IOP) (MUCH TIME PASSES)

MID-DILATION = PUPILLARY BLOCK
∡ CLOSES ← ↑ IOP ↵
POST CHAMBER

IRIS COVERS
OUTFLOW
↳ ↑ IOP → PAIN, BLURRY,
ALL CHAMBER FIXED MID-DILATION

VISION LOSS ←→ LASER
IRIDOTOMY

OPEN ∡ GLAUCOMA

PATH : IDIOPATHIC ↑ IOP
PRESSURE COMPROMISES
AXONS OF OPTIC N.

PT : INSIDIOUS ONSET OF
VISION LOSS

DX : SCREENING ↑ IOP
+ ↑ CUP-TO-DISC RATIO

TX : ↓ HUMOR   ↑ HUMOR
PRODUCTION   DRAINAGE
(CILIARY PROCESS) (UVEOSCLERAL)
α₂ – BRIMONIDINE – α₁
β-BLOCKER – TIMOLOL   PROSTAGLANDIN-PROST
DORZOLAMIDE CARBONIC ANHYDRASE-I   RHO KINASE

FUNDOSCOPIC △S

AGE-RELATED MACULAR DEGEN
LOSS OF CENTRAL VISION

WET = NEOVASCULARIZATION VEGF-I
DRY = DRUSEN DEPOSITS   LASER

CENTRAL RETINA ARTERY OCC.
PAINLESS LOSS OF MONOCULAR VISION
AMAUROSIS FUGAX (TIA)
RETINA WHITE, MACULA OBVIOUS
NO OTHER FND
↳ CVD IS SAME x̄
HEMORRHAGES   +   PROCOAGULABLE
ENGORGED VEINS   STATE

RETINAL DETACHMENT
PAINFULL MONOCULAR LOSS
"VEIL," PREVIOUS "FLOATERS"
HTN EMERGENCY, DECELERATION

PAPILLEDEMA
↑ IOP PUSHES OPTIC NERVE INTO
RETINA, LIFTING THE DISC INTO VITREOUS

HTN + DM FINDINGS
· COTTONWOOL SPOTS
· NEOVASCULARIZATION
· HEMORRHAGE

RETINITIS PIGMENTOSA
PROGRESSIVE BLINDNESS

The Ear—Audition and Balance

ANATOMY

① OUTER EAR: AUDITION "ONLY"
· PINNA DIRECTS SOUND. CARTILAGE TO BONE
· EXTERNAL AUDITORY MEATUS, CERUMEN
· HAIR-BEARING, KERATINIZED SSE (SKIN)

② MIDDLE EAR = AUDITION "ONLY"
TYMPANIC CAVITY = RESPIRATORY EPITHELIUM
AUDITORY CANAL EQUALIZES PRESSURE
MALLEUS TENSOR TYMPANI M TYMPANIC MEMBRANE
INCUS: "THE OTHER ONE!"
STAPES: STAPEDIUS M, OVAL "WINDOW"
(MEMBRANE)

③ INNER EAR
· VESTIBULE = BALANCE   VESTIBULO-
· COCHLEA = AUDITION   COCHLEAR
· WITHIN TEMPORAL BONE   N.

HAIR CELLS IN ENDOLYMPH

ENDOLYMPH: K⁺ 160   NA₋ CA₋
POTASSIUM CHANNELS DEPOLARIZE
STEREOCILIA – OPEN OR CLOSE

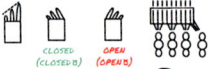

CLOSED   OPEN
(CLOSED ⊟) (OPEN ⊟)

FREQUENCY |||| |||||||| | | |

HEARING/COCHLEA

· SCALAS: TYMPANI (TYMPANIC)
(DUCTS) MEDIA (COCHLEAR)
VESTIBULI (VESTIBULAR)
· ORGAN OF CORTI
↳ BASILAR MEMBRANE
(WIGGLE DA BUTT)
↳ TECTORIAL MEMBRANE
(HOLDS HAIR STILL)
↳ INNER HAIR CELL IS
BATHED IN ENDOLYMPH
↳ WAY MORE STUFF
· AUDITORY REFLEX
↳ STAPEDIUS M. + ROUND "WINDOW"
GOES TAUT
↳ TENSOR TYMPANI M + TYMPANIC
MEMBRANE GOES TAUT

WEBER + RINNE TEST

① WEBER = LOCALIZATION
SOFTER + BROKEN

② RINNE = CONDUCTIVE
OR SENSORINEURAL

BONE > AIR = CONDUCTION
AIR > BONE = SENSORINEURAL

HEARING LOSS – CONDUCTIVE

① CERUMEN IMPACTION
Ø FEVER, REMOVE 7 OTOSCOPE

② OTITIS MEDIA
⊕ FEVER ⊕ PAIN, Ø 7 PINNA TUG
PNEUMATIC INSUFFLATION
RESP ABX → AMOX – CLAV

③ CHOLESTEATOMA
NON-KERA SQUAMOUS STRATIFIED
ERODES OSSICLES SURGICAL REMOVAL

④ OTHER: OTOSCLEROSIS, PAGET'S (ELDERLY)
OSTEOPETROSIS (CONGENITAL)

BALANCE
– KINOCILIA
– GEL

① ROTATIONAL PERCEPTION
· HAIR CELLS IN GEL 7 ROCKS
· SEMICIRCULAR CANALS
· CUPULA W/I AMPULLA
· X, Y, Z PLANES + FULL SPECTRUM
· MOVEMENT MOVES ENDOLYMPH,
ENDOLYMPH MOVES CUPULA

② DECELERATION/ACCELERATION
· HAIR CELLS IN GEL 7 ROCKS
· SACCULE, UTRICLE CALCIUM
· OTOCONIA   CARBONATE
· OTOLITH
· ACCELERATION/GRAVITY MOVE ROCKS
· ROCKS MOVE THE GEL

HEARING LOSS – SENSORINEURAL

① PRESBYCUSIS   – (BASS)
AGE → ↑ HIGH FREQUENCY HEARING
TINNITUS, CROWDED PLACES WORST
HEARING AIDS

② NOISE – INDUCED
↑ DB → ↓ HIGH FREQUENCY HEARING
SAA PREVENT 7 EAR PRO

③ OTOTOXIC DRUGS
LOOP DIURETIC TOO MUCH TOO FAST.
CISPLATIN, AMINOGLYCOSIDE

④ OTHER: STROKE, CRANIAL CANCER
(AICA)

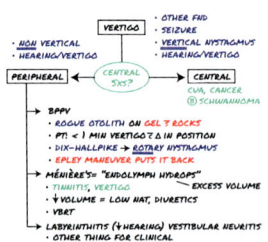

· OTHER FND
· SEIZURE
VERTIGO   · VERTICAL NYSTAGMUS
· NON VERTICAL   · HEARING/VERTIGO
· HEARING/VERTIGO
PERIPHERAL   CENTRAL   CENTRAL
5X5?   CVA, CANCER
⊗ SCHWANNOMA

↳ BPPV
· ROGUE OTOLITH ON GEL 7 ROCKS
· PT → < 1 MIN VERTIGO △ IN POSITION
· DIX-HALLPIKE → ROTARY NYSTAGMUS
· EPLEY MANEUVER PUTS IT BACK
↳ MÉNIÈRE's "ENDOLYMPH HYDROPS"
· TINNITIS, VERTIGO   EXCESS VOLUME
· ↓ VOLUME = LOW NAT, DIURETICS
· VBRT
↳ LABRINTHITIS (↓ HEARING) VESTIBULAR NEURITIS
· OTHER THING FOR CLINICAL

© 2021 OnlineMedEd

Neuroscience

Normal Testis

EMBRYOLOGY LITE

Wolffian Mesonephric Duct
Para Müllerian Ducts
Urogenital Sinus
Indifferent Gonad
Cortex Medulla
Ejaculator Duct → Urethra
Seminal Vesicles
Ductus Deferens
Head — Tunica Albuginea
Body — Tunica Vaginalis
Tail — Peritesticular Cavity — Ductus Deferens
BV — Tunica Vasculosa

DUCTS + HISTO

Epididymal Duct
Efferent Ducts
Rete Testis
Straight Tubules
Seminiferous Tubules
Complicated
Simple Cuboid
Pseudostratified Columnar +/- Stereocilia → Nuture Spermatozoa
Head — Convoluted No Lamina Propria Smooth Muscle
Tail (Stored) — Not Convoluted Ø Stereocilia Lots Of Smooth Muscle

ENDOCRINE

[HYPO]
G₊ ↓ GNRH
ANT PIT
LH ↑ G₊ ↓ FSH
Inhibin B
Leydig — Sertoli
Testosterone — Spermato-spermio-
Anti-Müllerian Hormone (AMH)
Androgen Binding Protein (ABP) ↳ Local Regulation
Systemic Testerone Regulation

VASCULATURE
Myoid ↑ Contractile
(R) Testicular Vein (IVC) 34° (L) Testicular Vein (renal)
FSH · LH ·
Convoluted Artery Pampiniform Plexus
CT

IMMUNITY SHIELD
Sertoli Cytoplasmic Barrier
Blood-Testis Barrier
Apical Compartment
FSH
Basal Compartment
Zona Occludens
Zona Adherens
E-Cadherins
Fenestrated

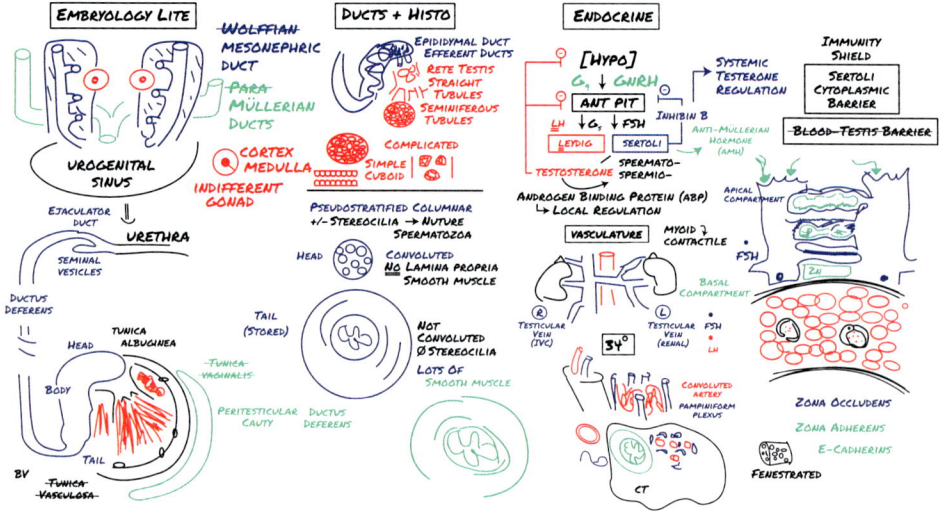

Sexual Differentiation Inside and Out

SEXUAL DIFFERENTIATION = 4 INDEPENDENT EVENTS

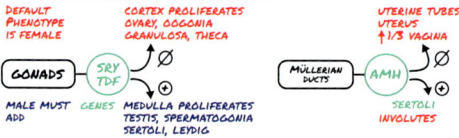

Default Phenotype Is Female
Cortex Proliferates Ovary, Oogonia Granulosa, Theca
Uterine Tubes Uterus ↑1/3 Vagina
GONADS — SRY TDF
Male Must Add Genes
Medulla Proliferates Testis, Spermatogonia Sertoli, Leydig
Müllerian Ducts — AMH
Sertoli Involutes

DISORDERS OF SEXUAL DIFFERENTIATION = DSD

DISORDER	GONADS (SRY TDF)	MÜLLERIAN (AMH)	MESONEPHRIC (TESTOSTERONE)	EXT GEN (5DHT)
5α-Reductase Deficiency (46,XY)	⊕ Testis	Involute	⊕ Male Tubes	✗ Female
Complete AIS (46,XY)	⊕ Testis	✗ Involute = No Tubes	✗ Involute	✗ Female
Gonadal Agenesis (46,XY) (45,XO)	✗ Streaks	✗ Female	✗ Involute	✗ Female
CAH (46,XY)	⊕ Testis	⊕ Involute	⊕ Male Tubes	⊕ Male = ØDSD
CAH (46,XX)	✗ Ovaries	✗ Female Tubes	✗ Involute	✗ Female Phenotype → DHEA → Masculinization

GONADS, F TUBES, M TUBES, EXT GENITALIA

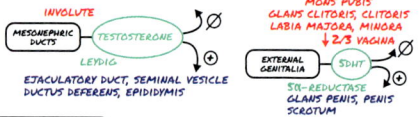

Mesonephric Ducts — Testosterone — Ø
Leydig
Ejaculatory Duct, Seminal Vesicle Ductus Deferens, Epididymis

Mons Pubis Glans Clitoris, Clitoris Labia Majora, Minora ↓2/3 Vagina
External Genitalia — 5DHT
5α-Reductase Glans Penis, Penis Scrotum

GERM CELLS

1. Gonadal Ridge On Urogenital Ridge
2. Mesoderm Proliferate Ridge To Bulge
3. Mesothelium Proliferate Into The Bulge (Sex-Cord)
4. Primordial Germ Cells Migrate Yolk Sac (Endodermal)

Cloaca — Urogenital Fold — Labiosacral Swelling — Genital Tubercle

DETAILS OF EXT GEN

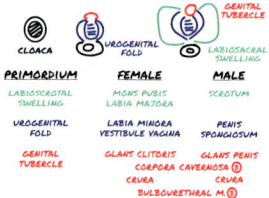

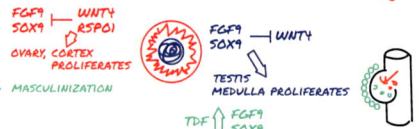

PRIMORDIUM	FEMALE	MALE
Labioscrotal Swelling	Mons Pubis Labia Majora	Scrotum
Urogenital Fold	Labia Minora Vestibule Vagina	Penis Spongiosum
Genital Tubercle	Glans Clitoris Corpora Cavernosa ⓑ Crura	Glans Penis Corpora Cavernosa ⓑ Crura Bulbourethral M. ⓑ

FGF9 SOX9 — WNT4 RSPO1
Ovary, Cortex Proliferates
FGF9 SOX9 — WNT4
Testis Medulla Proliferates
TDF ⇧ FGF9 SOX9

NOTES

Scrotal Pathologies

PAINLESS SWELLING

TRANSILLUMINATE = FLUID = SEE LIGHT
VALSALVA = LARGER/WORSE

↳ HYDROCELE = PERITESTICULAR CAVITY
- ⊕ TRANSILLUMINATION, ∅ VALSALVA
- INFANTILE→INDIRECT HERNIAS
- ADULT→ U.S. IATROGENIC, HERNIAS
  3RD→ W. BANCROFTI, CHLA (L)
UNIFORM SWELLING
DX: U/S FNA DRAIN
TX: SURGERY

↳ SPERMATOCELE = EPIDYMAL CYSTS
- ⊕ TRANSILLUMINATE, ∅ VALSAVA
- HEAD OF EPIDIDYMIS
- NONUNIFORM - POSTERIOR, SUPERIOR
DX: U/S FNA DRAIN
TX: SURGERY

↳ VARICOCELE = PAMPINIFORM PLEXUS
- ⊘ TRANSILLUMINATE, ↑ ∠ VALSALVA
- BAG OF WORMS
- Ⓛ SIDE, Ⓛ TESTICULAR → Ⓛ RENAL
  VEIN   VEIN
- NEW, ABRUPT ONSET, OLD MAN, SMOKE
  ↳ RCC, OCCLUDE/THROMBOSE
  DX: U/S

  TX: ABLATE   TX: UNDERLYING CAUSE
↳ HERNIA

PAINFUL SWELLING

PREHN'S SIGN = ↓ PAIN ∠ LIFT
CREMASTERIC REFLEX = LIFT ∠ STROKE
↳ EPIDIDYMITIS = EPIDIDYMIS
- ⊕ PREHN'S ⊕ CREMASTERIC
- TENDER POSTERIOR + SUPERIOR TESTIS
- STI GC/CHLA, YOUNG MALE
  SEXUALLY ACTIVE
  U/A, UCX, GC/CHLA → ABX
- UTI E. COLI, OLD MALE BPH
  U/A, UCX ——→ ABX
DX : ↑ ECHOES ↑ VASCULARITY

↳ ORCHITIS = TESTIS-ITIS
- ⊕ PREHN'S ⊖ CREMASTERIC
- MUMPS - UNVACCINATED, ≥ 10 YRS,
  PAROTITIS, ORCHITIS, FIBROSIS
  PUBERTY + FERTILITY PROBLEMS
- AUTOIMMUNE ORCHITIS 2/2 VASECTOMY
  GRANULOMATOUS (MNGC) FOREIGN
  BODIES

↳ TESTICULAR TORSION = ISCHEMIA
- ⊖ PREHN'S ⊖ CREMASTERIC REFLEX
PATH: TESTIS SPIN, ∅ TACKED DOWN, KINK
  VEINS (LOW-PRESSURE) ARTERY BLOOD IN
  UNDESCENDED TESTIS, PERITESTICULAR
  CAVITY
PT: ADOLESCENT, SUDDEN ONSET, 3 PROVOCATION
  SCROTAL POOP
DX: U/S ∠ DOPPLER = WHIRLPOOL, ∅ VASCULARITY
TX: SURGERY
  PINKS = Ⓑ ORCHIPEXY
  NOT = ORCHIECTOMY + ORCHIOPEXY
F/U: FERTILITY, PUBERTY, +/- STEROID

CANCER IN SCROTUM

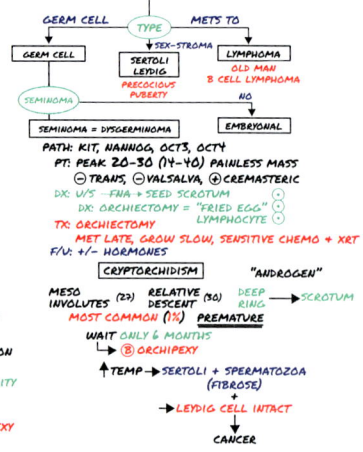

GERM CELL ── (TYPE) ── METS TO
         ↘ SEX-STROMA
GERM CELL   SERTOLI   LYMPHOMA
                 LEYDIG   OLD MAN
          SEMINOMA PRECOCIOUS B CELL LYMPHOMA
                    PUBERTY
                             NO
SEMINOMA = DYSGERMINOMA   EMBRYONAL
PATH: KIT, NANNOG, OCT3, OCT4
PT: PEAK 20-30 (14-40) PAINLESS MASS
  ⊖ TRANS, ⊖ VALSALVA ⊕ CREMASTERIC
DX: U/S FNA + SEED SCROTUM
  DX: ORCHIECTOMY = "FRIED EGG" ⊕
                   LYMPHOCYTE ⊕
TX: ORCHIECTOMY
  MET LATE, GROW SLOW, SENSITIVE CHEMO & XRT
F/U: +/- HORMONES

CRYPTORCHIDISM   "ANDROGEN"

MESO   (22) RELATIVE (30) DEEP ──→ SCROTUM
INVOLUTES   DESCENT   RING
  MOST COMMON (1%) PREMATURE
  WAIT ONLY 6 MONTHS
      ↳ ⊕ ORCHIPEXY
  ↑ TEMP → SERTOLI + SPERMATOZOA
                  (FIBROSE)
              +
          → LEYDIG CELL INTACT

              CANCER

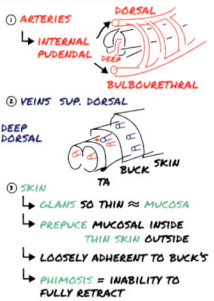

Erection and Ejaculation

SPERMATOGENESIS
① TYPE A (DARK) RESERVE
  STEM CELL. 2N. RARELY
② TYPE A (PALE) RENEWING
  STEM CELL. 2N. REGULAR
③ TYPE B UNDERGOES MANY
  MITOSIS UNTIL ALL...
④ 1° SPERMATOCYTE REPLICATES
  DNA (4N) THEN MEIOSIS 1
⑤ 2° SPERMATOCYTES DON'T
  REPLICATE, MEIOSIS 2
⑥ SPERMATIDS

SPERMIOGENESIS

SPERMATID   SPERMATOZOON
- ACROSOMAL CAP
  HEAD = 1N NUCLEUS
  NECK
- MIDPIECE
  MITOCHONDRIA
- TAIL = FLAGELLUM

DUCT HISTOLOGY
↳ DUCTUS DEFERENS

  INNER
  MIDDLE } MUSCLE
  OUTER
PSEUDOSTRATIFIED
COLUMNAR +/- STEREOCILIA

↳ SEMINAL VESICLE
  PSC ∠ PAPILLAE
MAKES
SEMEN LUMEN   LUMEN
WHITE
        PAPILLAE
        PAPILLAE

↳ PROSTATE GLAND
  FRUCTOSE, PSA, SEE RENAL

SQUAMOUS CELL CARCINOMA
BLUE = WAFER THIN
       KERATIN
GREEN = NO KERATIN
WHERE HPV 16, 18
CAN INFECT
AND CAUSE CANCER
ALSO POVERTY + INF XNS

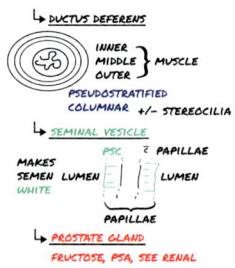

PENIS HISTOLOGY
LAYERS: SKIN (COLLES)
  BUCK'S   * PEYRONIE'S
  TUNICA   EXCESS
  ALBUGINEA   FIBROUS
  CORPORA   GIVES
  CAVERNOSA   PAINFUL
URETHRA CORPUS   CURVE
         SPONGIOSUM

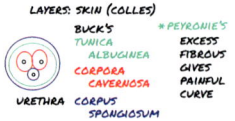

PENIS ANATOMY + VASC
① ARTERIES   DORSAL
  ↳ INTERNAL
    PUDENDAL   DEEP
                 BULBOURETHRAL
② VEINS SUP. DORSAL
DEEP
DORSAL
              BUCK SKIN
              TA
③ SKIN
  ↳ GLANS SO THIN ≈ MUCOSA
  ↳ PREPUCE MUCOSAL INSIDE
         THIN SKIN OUTSIDE
  ↳ LOOSELY ADHERENT TO BUCK'S
  ↳ PHIMOSIS = INABILITY TO
    FULLY RETRACT

ERECTION + EJACULATION
"POINT THEN SHOOT"
       OR
"DILATE ARTERIOLES"
      AND
"CONTRACT α"

* PNS
  ERECTION = DILATE SPHICTERS
  = SPECIFICALLY OF ARTERIOLES
  NO = ↑cGMP = DILATION
  CORPORA ENGORGE, HELICINE STRETCH,
  VEINS COLLAPSE = ERECTION
                   ACHIEVED

* SNS
  EJACULATION = CONTRACT VIA α
- COORDINATED PERISTALSIS
  FROM TAIL OF EPIDIDYMIS
  THROUGH URETHRA VIA
  BULBOURETHRAL MUSCLES
- CLOSURE OF URETHRAL VALVE
  BLOCKING PATH TO BLADDER
- EJECTION @ HIGH
  VELOCITY

N O T E S

The Healthy Ovary

OVARY
1. GERMINAL EPITHELIUM PERITONEUM
2. TUNICA ALBUGINEA
3. FOLLICLES
4. STROMA

BV, LYMPH, NERVES

AXIS INDEPENDENT
AXIS DEPENDENT

FOLLICLES
1. PRIMORDIAL FOLLICLES = OOCYTE + SIMPLE SQUAMOUS — GRANULOSA
2. EARLY PRIMARY " + SIMPLE CUBOID *
3. LATE PRIMARY " + ZP + STRATIFIED CUBOID * SIMPLE COLUMNAR
4. EARLY SECONDARY ANTRUM + THECA FOLLICULI
5. LATE SECONDARY ADD CUMULUS OOPHORUS
6. MATURE ADD SIZE
CORONA RADIATA

MEIOSIS 1   MEIOSIS 2

THE AXIS
?
HYPOTHALAMUS — IMPROVE PULSATILITY
PULSATILE | GnRH
GONADOTROPES
LH / FSH ↑GnRH-R ↓FSH
THECA | GRANULOSA ↑LH-R
ANDROGEN + AROMATASE = ESTROGEN
PROGESTERONE STEROID GENE TRANSCRIPTION
STEROID HORMONE INFLUENCE GENE TRANSCRIPTION

LH SURGE

CORPUS LUTEUM
↳ LUTEINIZED
LH-R

PROGESTERONE
LH-R = HCG-R
PHCG

OVARIAN LIG + VASC
(R)   (L)
"VARICOCELE"
SUSPENSORY LIGAMENT OF OVARY "TORSION"
OVARIAN LIGAMENT → FIBROUS
OVARY

OVARIAN CYCLE
FOLLICULAR | LUTEAL
ESTROGEN | PROGESTERONE
OVULATION
ALL ACTIVE FOLLICLES | ONE FOLLICLE CORPUS LUTEUM
FEED FORWARD THE AXIS | SILENCES THE AXIS
PROMOTE OVULATION | INHIBIT OVULATION

HIGH FSH   WANE FSH   NO FSH

LH
FSH
ESTROGEN
PROGESTERONE

HYPO — GnRH-R
ANT — FSH
FOLLICLES
OV
CLOSE
MED — FSH-R

→ OVULATE
→ BYE FELICIA!
→ QUIT
→ TRY AGAIN

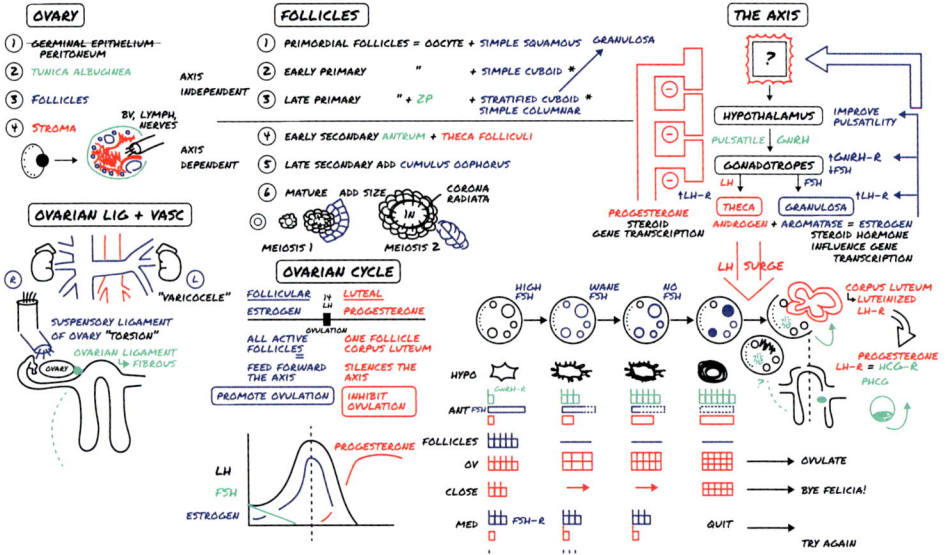

The Healthy Uterus

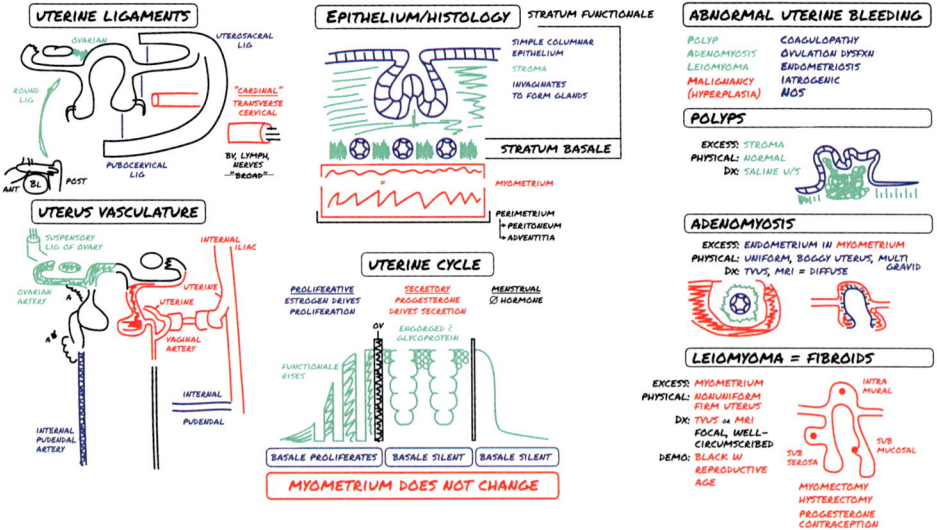

UTERINE LIGAMENTS
OVARIAN LIG
UTEROSACRAL LIG
ROUND LIG
"CARDINAL" TRANSVERSE CERVICAL
PUBOCERVICAL LIG
BV, LYMPH, NERVES "BROAD"
ANT | POST

UTERUS VASCULATURE
SUSPENSORY LIG OF OVARY
INTERNAL ILIAC
OVARIAN ARTERY
UTERINE
UTERINE ARTERY
VAGINAL ARTERY
INTERNAL
PUDENDAL
INTERNAL PUDENDAL ARTERY

EPITHELIUM/HISTOLOGY
STRATUM FUNCTIONALE
SIMPLE COLUMNAR EPITHELIUM
STROMA
INVAGINATES TO FORM GLANDS
STRATUM BASALE
MYOMETRIUM
PERIMETRIUM
→ PERITONEUM
→ ADVENTITIA

UTERINE CYCLE
PROLIFERATIVE | SECRETORY | MENSTRUAL
ESTROGEN DRIVES PROLIFERATION | PROGESTERONE DRIVES SECRETION | Ø HORMONE
OV
ENGORGED & GLYCOPROTEIN
FUNCTIONALE RISES

BASALE PROLIFERATES | BASALE SILENT | BASALE SILENT
MYOMETRIUM DOES NOT CHANGE

ABNORMAL UTERINE BLEEDING
POLYP | COAGULOPATHY
ADENOMYOSIS | OVULATION DYSFXN
LEIOMYOMA | ENDOMETRIOSIS
MALIGNANCY (HYPERPLASIA) | IATROGENIC
| NOS

POLYPS
EXCESS: STROMA
PHYSICAL: NORMAL
DX: SALINE U/S

ADENOMYOSIS
EXCESS: ENDOMETRIUM IN MYOMETRIUM
PHYSICAL: UNIFORM, BOGGY UTERUS, MULTI GRAVID
DX: TVUS, MRI = DIFFUSE

LEIOMYOMA = FIBROIDS
EXCESS: MYOMETRIUM
PHYSICAL: NONUNIFORM FIRM UTERUS
DX: TVUS or MRI FOCAL, WELL-CIRCUMSCRIBED
DEMO: BLACK W REPRODUCTIVE AGE
INTRA MURAL
SUB SEROSA
SUB MUCOSAL
MYOMECTOMY
HYSTERECTOMY
PROGESTERONE CONTRACEPTION

NOTES

Endometrial Hyperplasia and Carcinoma

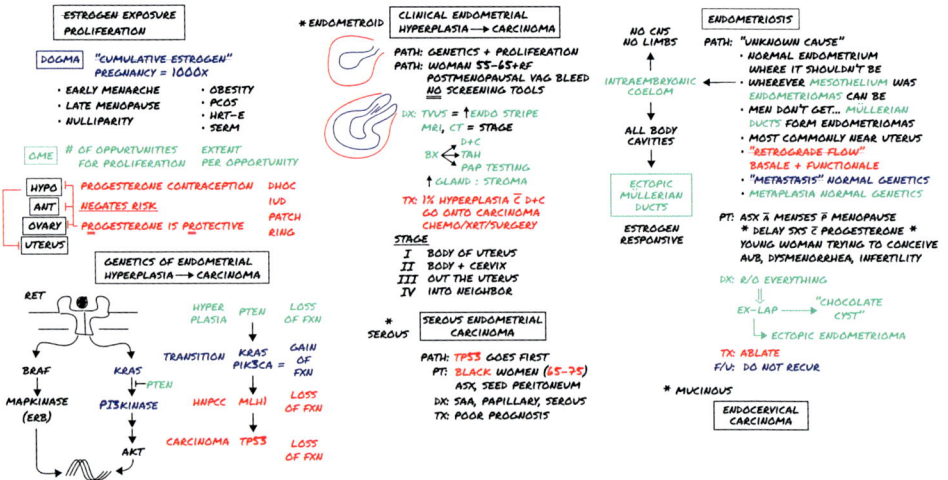

ESTROGEN EXPOSURE PROLIFERATION

DOGMA — "CUMULATIVE ESTROGEN" PREGNANCY = 1000×
- EARLY MENARCHE
- LATE MENOPAUSE
- NULLIPARITY
- OBESITY
- PCOS
- HRT-E
- SERM

OME — # OF OPPURTUNITIES FOR PROLIFERATION — EXTENT PER OPPORTUNITY

HYPO — PROGESTERONE CONTRACEPTION — DHOC
ANT — NEGATES RISK — IUD
OVARY — PROGESTERONE IS PROTECTIVE — PATCH
UTERUS — RING

GENETICS OF ENDOMETRIAL HYPERPLASIA → CARCINOMA

RET

HYPER PLASIA — PTEN — LOSS OF FXN

TRANSITION — KRAS PIK3CA = GAIN OF FXN

BRAF — KRAS — PTEN
MAPKINASE (ErB) — PI3KINASE — HNPCC MLH1 — LOSS OF FXN

AKT

CARCINOMA TP53 — LOSS OF FXN

* ENDOMETROID

CLINICAL ENDOMETRIAL HYPERPLASIA → CARCINOMA

PATH: GENETICS + PROLIFERATION
PATH: WOMAN 55-65+RF POSTMENOPAUSAL VAG BLEED NO SCREENING TOOLS

DX: TVUS = ↑ENDO STRIPE
MRI, CT = STAGE
D+C
BX — TAH
PAP TESTING
↑ GLAND : STROMA

TX: 1% HYPERPLASIA c̄ D+C
GO ONTO CARCINOMA
CHEMO/XRT/SURGERY

STAGE
I — BODY OF UTERUS
II — BODY + CERVIX
III — OUT THE UTERUS
IV — INTO NEIGHBOR

* SEROUS ENDOMETRIAL CARCINOMA

PATH: TP53 GOES FIRST
PT: BLACK WOMEN (65-75)
ASX, SEED PERITONEUM
DX: SAA, PAPILLARY, SEROUS
TX: POOR PROGNOSIS

NO CNS
NO LIMBS

INTRAEMBRYONIC COELOM

ALL BODY CAVITIES

ECTOPIC MULLERIAN DUCTS

ESTROGEN RESPONSIVE

ENDOMETRIOSIS

PATH: "UNKNOWN CAUSE"
- NORMAL ENDOMETRIUM WHERE IT SHOULDN'T BE
- WHEREVER MESOTHELIUM WAS ENDOMETRIOMAS CAN BE
- MEN DON'T GET... MULLERIAN DUCTS FORM ENDOMETRIOMAS
- MOST COMMONLY NEAR UTERUS
- "RETROGRADE FLOW" BASALE + FUNCTIONALE
- "METASTASIS" NORMAL GENETICS
- METAPLASIA NORMAL GENETICS

PT: ASX c̄ MENSES p̄ MENOPAUSE
* DELAY SXS c̄ PROGESTERONE *
YOUNG WOMAN TRYING TO CONCEIVE
AUB, DYSMENORRHEA, INFERTILITY

DX: R/O EVERYTHING
EX-LAP — "CHOCOLATE CYST"
↳ ECTOPIC ENDOMETRIOMA

TX: ABLATE
F/U: DO NOT RECUR

* MUCINOUS
ENDOCERVICAL CARCINOMA

Cervix and Vagina

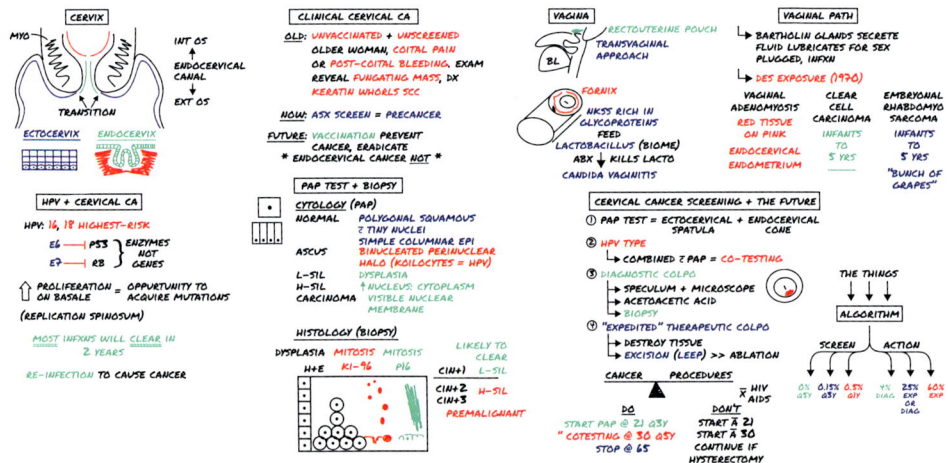

CERVIX

MYO
INT OS
ENDOCERVICAL CANAL
EXT OS
TRANSITION
ECTOCERVIX — ENDOCERVIX

HPV + CERVICAL CA

HPV: 16, 18 HIGHEST-RISK
E6 — P53 ENZYMES NOT GENES
E7 — RB

↑ PROLIFERATION = OPPURTUNITY TO
ON BASALE ACQUIRE MUTATIONS
(REPLICATION SPINOSUM)

MOST INFXNS WILL CLEAR IN 2 YEARS

RE-INFECTION TO CAUSE CANCER

CLINICAL CERVICAL CA

OLD: UNVACCINATED + UNSCREENED
OLDER WOMAN, COITAL PAIN
OR POST-COITAL BLEEDING. EXAM
REVEAL FUNGATING MASS, DX
KERATIN WHORLS SCC

NOW: ASX SCREEN = PRECANCER

FUTURE: VACCINATION PREVENT
CANCER, ERADICATE
* ENDOCERVICAL CANCER HOT *

PAP TEST + BIOPSY

CYTOLOGY (PAP)
NORMAL — POLYGONAL SQUAMOUS
c̄ TINY NUCLEI
SIMPLE COLUMNAR EPI
ASCUS — BINUCLEATED PERINUCLEAR
HALO (KOILOCYTES = HPV)
L-SIL — DYSPLASIA
H-SIL — ↑ NUCLEUS: CYTOPLASM
CARCINOMA — VISIBLE NUCLEAR
MEMBRANE

HISTOLOGY (BIOPSY)

DYSPLASIA — MITOSIS — MITOSIS — LIKELY TO CLEAR
H+E — KI-96 — P16 — CIN+1 — L-SIL
CIN+2 — H-SIL
CIN+3 — PREMALIGNANT

VAGINA

RECTOUTERINE POUCH
BL — TRANSVAGINAL APPROACH

FORNIX
NKSS RICH IN GLYCOPROTEINS
FEED LACTOBACILLUS (BIOME)
ABX ↓ KILLS LACTO
CANDIDA VAGINITIS

VAGINAL PATH

↳ BARTHOLIN GLANDS SECRETE
FLUID LUBRICATES FOR SEX
PLUGGED, INFXN

↳ DES EXPOSURE (1970)

VAGINAL ADENOMYOSIS — CLEAR CELL CARCINOMA — EMBRYONAL RHABDOMYO SARCOMA
RED TISSUE ON PINK — INFANTS TO 5 YRS — INFANTS TO 5 YRS
ENDOCERVICAL ENDOMETRIUM — "BUNCH OF GRAPES"

CERVICAL CANCER SCREENING + THE FUTURE

① PAP TEST = ECTOCERVICAL + ENDOCERVICAL
SPATULA CONE
② HPV TYPE
↳ COMBINED c̄ PAP = CO-TESTING
③ DIAGNOSTIC COLPO
↳ SPECULUM + MICROSCOPE
↳ ACETOACETIC ACID
↳ BIOPSY
④ "EXPEDITED" THERAPEUTIC COLPO
↳ DESTROY TISSUE
↳ EXCISION (LEEP) >> ABLATION

CANCER — PROCEDURES

THE THINGS
↓ ↓ ↓
ALGORITHM
SCREEN — ACTION

DO — DON'T
" COTESTING @ 30 Q5Y — START c̄ 21 — START c̄ 30
START PAP @ 21 Q3Y — x̄ HIV AIDS — CONTINUE IF HYSTERECTOMY
STOP @ 65

0% 0.15% 0.5% — Y% 25% 60%
Q5Y Q3Y Q1Y — DIAG EXP OR DIAG EXP

NOTES

Fertilization, Implantation, and Early Embryogenesis

OnlineMedEd

CAPACITATION
1. Ca^{2+} CHANNELS HYPERMOTILITY (KICK HARDER)
2. ZP3 IS LIGAND (HOLD ON) FOR ZP-R
3. ACROSOMAL CAP EZYMES

FERTILIZATION
1. FUSION OF MEMBRANE
2. INJECTION OF HAPLOID NUCLEUS
3. SPERMATOZOON IP_3 INDUCES OOCYTE DEPOLARIZATION
   - CORTICAL RXN, ↑ZP SIZE
   - SPERMATOZOA STUNNED
   - CORONA RADIATA LETS GO (MEIOSIS 2 DISINHIBITED)
4. MEIOSIS 2 COMPLETES (POLAR BODY)
5. NUCLEI JOIN

MORULA
ZYGOTE → 2 → 4 → 8 → 16 → BLASTOCYST

$\overline{A}$ AMPULLA = ECTOPIC
$\overline{P}$ AMPULLA = MISSED

CELL ORGANIZATION
ZYGOTE CLEAVAGE

INNER CELL MASS → OUTER CELL MASS IS TROPHOBLAST
HYPOBLAST EPIBLAST → CYTOTROPHOBLAST
YOLK SAC AMNIOTIC CAVITY EMBRYO → SYNCYTIOTROPHOBLAST
FETUS EE + MESODERM → CHORION
AMNION NEONATE

IMPLANTATION
TROPHOBLAST: CYTOTROPHOBLASTS DIVIDE + DIFFERENTIATE ONE DAUGHTER TO BECOME SYNCYTIOTROPHOBLAST
∅ PLASMA MEMBRANE, MANY NUCLEI
ERODES ENDOMETRIUM SEARCH OF BV

HYPOBLAST: PROLIFERATES TO CONTROL BLASTOCYST CAVITY

EPIBLAST: PROVIDES THE EXTRAEMBRYONIC MESODERM THAT WILL BECOME BV OF PLACENTA
- AMNIOTIC CAVITY
EPIBLAST
- EMBRYO/TRILAMINAR/ETC

CHORIONIC CAVITY
TROPHOBLAST: CHORIONIC VILLI CHORIONIC PLATE
HYPOBLAST: ENDODERM TO EMBRYO (PRIMORDIAL GERM CELLS)
EPIBLAST: MORE EMBRYO
   MORE AMNION
   MORE EE MESODERM
EE MESODERM: CONNECTING STALK SOMATIC
   SPLANCHNIC EEM
   SOMATIC EEM +

PRIMITIVE STREAK FORWARD
TROPHOBLAST: CHORION, PLACENTA
EPIBLAST: AMNION, AMNIOTIC CAVITY/FLUID
HYPOBLAST: BYE FELICIA! (DISAPPEARS)
EE MESODERM: BVs OF CHORION CONNECTING STALK
   (PLACENTA) (UMBILICAL CORD)

MEMBRANES
CHORION
AMNION
HYPO-
ENDOMETRIAL
DECIDUA

CHORIONIC VILLI
PRIMARY: CYTOTROPHOBLAST
SECONDARY: MESODERM
TERTIARY: BVs

SPLANCHNIC
TWO DEOXYGENATED ARTERIES
OXYGENATED UMBILICAL VEIN
WHARTON'S JELLY

SYNCYTIO-TROPHOBLAST
VILLUS
NO MEMBRANE
NO ANTIGENS
MATERNAL BLOOD

Reproductive Endocrinology—Puberty, Menopause, and the HPO

HPA ? GH AXIS

HYPOTHAL
GnRH
ANT PIT
OVARIAN

ANDROGENS ESTROGEN
BREAST HAIR UTERUS
THELARCHE PUBARCHE MENARCHE

PUBERTY
NORMAL F: 8-13
   M: 9-14
THELARCHE → 3 YRS → MENARCHE
TANNER STAGE 1-5
- BREAST
- PUBIC HAIR
- AXILLARY HAIR
- GONAD SIZE (M)

ADRENARCHE: HPA AXIS
6-8 YRS OLD, INDEPENDENT UNNECESSARY FOR HPO AXIS

GH AXIS MAXIMAL GROWTH VELOCITY = MENARCHE

ONCE ON, IT DOES NOT TURN OFF

2° AMENORRHEA ∅ BLEED $\bar{P}$ MENSES
BABY ⊕UPT
H+P +FSH OVARIAN FAILURE W/S: FOLLICLES
UPT, TSH/T4, LH/FSH, PRL ↑PRL
   ↑FSH, LH PROLACTINEMIA ENDOCRINE
PROGESTIN CHALLENGE ⊕BLEED PCOS W/S: FOLLICLES
   ∅ BLEED AXIS

HYPO EXERCISE ANOREXIA STRESS
MRI ANT PIT PANHYPO PIT SHEEHAN'S APOPLEXY ARC
FSH RESISTANT OVARY PREMATURE OVARIAN FAILURE MENOPAUSE
OVARY ENDOCRINE PRO CHALLENGE ASHERMAN ABLATION
UTERUS ⊕UPT PREGNANCY

MENOPAUSE ∅ $\bar{P}$ 12 MONTHS
NORMAL AVG: 52 YRS
FOLLICLE DEPLETION
↓ESTROGEN
↑FSH, ↑LH, W/S = ∅ FOLLICLES
VASOMOTOR SXS (HOT FLASHES/FLUSHES)
VENLAFAXINE
→ MOOD SWINGS
OSTEOPOROSIS Ca^{2+}, VIT D
VAGINAL ATROPHY
↑HEART DZ
-ESTROGEN-

PCOS
F < 40 (POI)
PATH: UNKNOWN RESISTANCE INSULIN, FSH, CLT
PT: REPRODUCTIVE AGE, INFERTILITY OBESE, HIRSUTE, DIABETIC LH:FSH 3:1 (NORMAL)
DX: 1 POLYCYSTIC OVARIES (U/S)
   2 ANOVULATION (AUB, INFERTILITY)
   3 HYPERANDROGENISM (PHYSICAL, LABS)
TX: DESIRES FERTILITY / ∅
CLOMIPHENE METFORMIN
PULSATILE GnRH PROGESTIN CONTRACEPTION IUD

PRECOCIOUS PUBERTY = TOO SOON
DEFINED: F < 8, M < 9, ⊕ SEX 2° CHAR
PATH: EXCESS ESTROGEN

CENTRAL PERIPHERAL
HYPO ↓GnRH
ANT PIT ↓FSH/LH ↓FSH/LH
OVARY ↑ESTROGEN ↑ESTROGEN ↑ESTROGEN
   HYPOTHAL ANTPIT GRANULOSA-THECA
W/W: BONE AGE (X-RAY)
   LH LEVEL GnRH ANALOG LEUPROLIDE
CENTRAL PERIPHERAL
MRI BRAIN U/S OVARIES

DELAYED PUBERTY + 1° AMENORRHEA
PATH: DEFICIENT ESTROGEN 13, 15, OR 3 YRS

HYPOGONADOTROPIC HYPOGONADISM (CENTRAL) HYPERGONADOTROPIC HYPOGONADISM (PERIPHERAL)
DELAY HYPO KALLMANN (ANOSMIA)
FSH LH ANT PIT PANHYPOPIT
CENTRAL PERIPHERAL OVARY STREAK
GnRH STIM TEST HYPO ↑FSH L → 45,XO 47,XYY
↓∆ FSH ANT PIT MRI UTERUS MA CAIS

ANATOMY
EYES AXIS BREAST
W/S ANATOMY: UTERUS
BIMANUAL

⊕ ⊖
PREGNANT MULLERIAN
ANOREXIA AGENESIS
IMPERFORATE COMPLETE
HYMEN AIS
AXIS KALLMANN PANHYPO PIT CRANIO — STREAK

184

© 2021 OnlineMedEd

NOTES

Ovarian Cancers

IN GENERAL
1. MÜLLERIAN EPITHELIUM
2. GERM CELL
3. SEX-CORD STROMAL

MÜLLERIAN SEVERITY
1. BENIGN
2. BORDERLINE
3. MALIGNANT

ADNEXAL MASS

BENIGN	MALIGNANT
< 10 CM	≥ 10 CM
UNILOCULAR	LOCULATIONS
FLUID	SOLID
THIN-WALL	THICK-WALL
Ø DOPPLER	⊕ DOPPLER

RISK FOR MÜLLERIAN
"CUMULATIVE-ESTROGEN"
EARLY MENARCHE	OBESITY
LATE MENOPAUSE	PCOS
NULLIPARITY	HRT-E
	SERM

↑ PROLIFERATION = ↑ MUTATIONS
PROGESTERONE CONTRACEPTION
NEGATES RISK
· BRCA1/2

```
        12                    52
     MENARCHE             MENOPAUSE
  ___|_____|___
GERM CELL    BENIGN         MALIGNANT
STROMAL     MÜLLERIAN       MÜLLERIAN
```

MÜLLERIAN EPITHELIAL OVARIAN CANCER
↳ SEROUS CYSTADENO(MA, CARCINOMA)
- SEROUS FLUID WITHIN CYST
- UTERINE TUBE EPITHELIUM
  PAPILLAE, COLUMNAR EPI
  c̄ CILIA
- KRAS, PIK3CA LOW GRADE
  TP53, BRCA   HIGH GRADE
- MULTICYSTIC SPACES THAT
  BECOME MORE SOLID AS
  DZ ADVANCES

↳ MUCINOUS CYSTADENO(MA, CARCINOMA)
- MUCINOUS FLUID WITHIN CYSTS
- ENDOCERVICAL ENDOMETRIUM
- KRAS MOST COMMON
- COLUMNAR s̄ CILIA +
  GLYCOPROTEINS
- DIFFERENT STAGES EVEN
  ON PAPILLAE

↳ ENDOMETROID
- NO CYSTS, NO FLUID
- ENDOMETRIOSIS
- ENDOMETRIAL EPITHELIUM
- PTEN, PIK3CA, KRAS
  + β-CATENIN
  TP53 = MALIGNANT

GERM CELL
↳ DYSGERMINOMA
- FEMALE SEMINOMA
- KIT, NANNOG, OCT3/4
- FRIED-EGG HISTOLOGY
- INVADE LATE, GROW SLOW
  SENSITIVE CHEMO/XRT
- CHILDHOOD

↳ YOLK SAC, ENDODERMAL SINUS
- PRODUCES AFP
- TYPICALLY UNILATERAL
  AND YOUNG WOMEN
- SCHILLER-DUVAL, "GLOMERULOID"

↳ CHORIOCARCINOMA
- MOLAR PREGNANCIES
- CYTO, SYNCYTIOTROPHOBLASTS
- SECRETES hCG

↳ TERATOMA, DERMOID CYST
- BENIGN IN GIRLS (MATURE)
  MALIGNANT IN BOYS (IMMATURE)
- 3 GERM LAYERS, MC
  SKIN, HAIR, TEETH
- GET ENORMOUS
  WEIGHT GAIN DESPITE EXERCISE
  OVARIAN TORSION

SEX CORD STROMAL
↳ PURE GRANULOSA
- ESTROGEN SECRETING CAUSE
  PRECOCIOUS PUBERTY (GIRLS)
  FEMINIZATION (BREAST, BOYS)
- INHIBIN B TRACK REMISSION
- HISTO: CALL-EXNER · FOXL
- ↑ ESTROGEN = FEMALE CANCER

↳ SERTOLI-LEYDIG
- TESTOSTERONE SECRETING CAUSES
  PRECOCIOUS PUBERTY (BOYS)
  MASCULINIZATION (GIRLS)
- HISTO: REINKE CRYSTALS W/I LEYDIG
- MORE COMMON IN GIRLS
- DICER1

↳ FIBROTHECOMA
- NO HORMONE
- FIBROBLASTS COULD BECOME THECA CELLS
- MEIG'S SYNDROME = ASCITES
- HYDROTHORAX, THECOMA RESOLVES
  p̄ RESECTION OF THECOMA

⟹ STRUMA OVARII
TERATOMA PRODUCES T4
HYPERTHYROIDISM, COL + RAIU

CARCINOID
TERATOMA SEROTONIN
FLUSHING, WHEEZING, DIARRHEA
(R) ♡ VALVE

The Healthy Breast

ANATOMY
DERMIS
EPIDERMIS
AREOLA
NIPPLE
SUB Q
AXILLARY LN
↓ DENSE = UPPER OUTER QUADRANT
LACTIFEROUS DUCTS 12-20
COMBINED = MAMMARY GLAND
INTERLOBULAR STROMA
LACTIFEROUS DUCTS

TDLU, HISTOLOGY
SIMPLE COLUMNAR ACINAR CELLS
SIMPLE CUBOID DUCT-LINING

INTRALOBULAR = LOOSE CONNECTIVE TISSUE STROMA
LOBULE
INTRA LOBULAR DUCTULE
INTERLOBULAR STROMA (ADIPOSE)
INTERLOBULAR DUCTS
DENSE CONNECTIVE TISSUE

PREGNANCY
1ST TRI: PROLIFERATION DUCTULES
ESTROGEN
2ND TRI: ACINI PROLIFERATE (BREAST ENLARGE)
3RD TRI: DIFFERENTIATION TDLU
PROGESTERONE
↳ HYPO   x [HYPO]
DOPAMINE ⊣ ⊖
ANT PIT   DELIVERY ⟹ (ANT PIT)

DEVELOPMENT
- DEFAULT PHENOTYPE IS NOTHING
  ESTROGEN ⊕
OVARY → ADULT
INFANT
TESTIS → TESTOSTERONE ⊕
· MILK LINES (ECTOPIC)
· CHILDHOOD: LACTIFEROUS DUCTS, DENSE STROMA (DERMIS)
· REPRODUCTIVE YEARS: LACTIFEROUS DUCTS, STROMA, ADIPOSE, LOBULES, FEW ACINI
· PREGNANT: LOBULES, MANY ACINI, LACT. DUCTS, STROMA, ADIPOSE
· POSTMENOPAUSE: LACTIFEROUS SINUS, ADIPOSE

BREAST MILK AXIS
HYPOTHAL
⊣ DOPAMINE
POST PIT ⊕
GONADOTROPES ⊖
LACTOTROPES
OXYTOCIN (FEED)
FSH, LH | GNRH-R
OVARIES
PROLACTIN
(14 DAYS)
NO CYCLES
MAMMARY GLAND
MYOEPITHELIAL CELLS
SINUS DUCT
MILK IN LOBULES
MILK IN SINUS
SUCKLING
MILK LETDOWN REFLEX
MILK IN BABY

BREAST MILK HISTOLOGY
ACINAR
SIMPLE COLUMNAR
c̄ MICROVILLI
"ALVEOLI" SAME

BREAST MILK
LACTALBUMIN
CASEIN
LACTOSE
LIPID AGGREGATES
WATER, IONS
IgA, IgG
~ 500 CALORIES/DAY

H₂O   IONS

NOTES

Breast Pathologies Not Cancer

OnlineMedEd

NOT MASSES

↳ **FAT NECROSIS**
TRAUMA ADIPOSE = SAPONIFICATION
BREAST BX ⟹ CALCIFICATION
BREAST CANCER ⟹
COMPROMISE MAMMOGRAM

↳ **MASTITIS**
OBSTRUCTION OF ONE LACT DUCT
  IN YOUNG FEMALE BREASTFEEDING
ASYMMETRIC + NONUNIFORM REDNESS,
  FLUCTUANCE, TENDER
BREASTFEED, BABY-SAFE
  ANTI-STAPH (DICLOX)

↳ **GYNECOMASTIA**
• MEN NOTICE MORE
• ↑ BREAST TISSUE
ASYMMETRIC + NONUNIFORM + ⓑ
↓ ESTROGEN OR ↓ ANTI-ANDROGENS
CIRRHOSIS : GnRH : FLUTAMIDE
  5α-I : FINASTERIDE

EPLERENONE ← ALDOSTERONE

↳ KETOCONAZOLE   CIMETIDINE
  (POWDER)   (NOT A CLASS
                   EFFECT)

↳ **GALACTORRHEA**

FIBROADENOMA

PATH: PROLIFERATION OF STROMA
  ESTROGEN-RESPONSIVE
PT: PREMENOPAUSAL WOMEN
  FIRM, SLOWLY-GROWING MASS
  WELL-DEMARCATED, MOBILE
  WILL NOT REGRESS
DX: MAMMOGRAM ⎤ WELL
  U/S BX ⎦ CIRCUMSCRIBED
    ↳ ↑STROMA : GLAND
TX: ANOVULATORY CONTRACEPTION
  SURGERY
  WAIT FOR MENOPAUSE

PHYLLODES TUMOR

PATH: PROLIFERATION OF STROMA
  AGGRESIVE + E-INDEPENDENT
PT: POSTMENOPAUSAL WOMAN
  FAST-GROWING, FIRM
  WELL-DEMARCATED, MOBILE
DX: MAMMOGRAM ⎤ WELL
  U/S BX ⎦ CIRCUMSCRIBED
    ↳ LEAF-LIKE PROJECTIONS
      CLEFTS OF STROMA
      "LINED" BY EPITHELIUM
      CUBOID COLUMNAR
TX: RESECTION

FIBROCYSTIC △

PATH: PROLIFERATION TDLU
  ESTROGEN-RESPONSIVE
PT: PREMENOPAUSAL WOMEN
  MASSES, PREMENSTRUAL
  PAIN, LUMPS + BUMPS
  THAT REGRESS + MIGRATE
⑧ ASYMMETRIC, NONUNIFORM
  NORMAL, Ø TX

U/S → FNA
↳ **CYSTS**
△ DUCT SIZE 2/2
DUCTS FILLING ⊃
BLUE-BROWN FLUID
BLUE-DOMED CYSTS

* **MAMMOGRAM**
↳ **ADENOSIS**
↑ # ACINI/LOBULE
FOCAL, NONUNIFORM
HISTOLOGY
CALCIFICATIONS

* **PHYSICAL**
↳ **FIBROSIS**
NORMAL FIBROBLASTS
COLLAGEN
NODULAR △S, FIRM
PERMANENT

PROLIFERATION OF DUCTS + ACINI ☉̄ ATYPIA

↳ **INTRADUCTAL PAPILLOMA**
LACTIFEROUS DUCT
ⓤ NIPPLE DISCHARGE
PROLIFERATIVE TYPE
PAPILLARY GROWTH
CONNECTING STALK

↳ **EPITHELIAL HYPERPLASIA**
CUBOID OR COLUMNAR
PROLIFERATIVE TYPE
EPITHELIAL STACKING
ASSOCIATED
APOCRINE METAPLASIA

↳ **SCLEROSING ADENOSIS**
↑ # ACINI/LOBULE
NONUNIFORM, FOCAL, SCARRING
CALCIFICATIONS, NODULAR △S
• Ø CENTRAL NIDUS
• Ø RADIAL SCAR

+ COMPLEX
• CENTRAL NIDUS
• RADIAL SCAR

PROLIFERATION OF DUCTS + ACINI ⊂̄ ATYPIA

ATYPICAL HYPERPLASIA		CARCINOMA IN SITU			INVASIVE CARCINOMA	
⊕ ATYPIA	→	⊕ ATYPIA			⊕ ATYPIA	CELLS INTO
DUCTS NOT FILLED		DUCTS FILLED			DUCTS FILLED	STROMA...
⊕ BM INTACT		⊕ BM INTACT			BM INVADED	
ATYPICAL LOBULAR HYPERPLASIA	E-CADHERIN GENES	LOBULAR (LCIS) ⊕ CALCIFICATIONS			INVASIVE LOBULAR CARCINOMA	SINGLE LINES INDIVIDUAL Ø DESMOPLASTIC
ATYPICAL DUCTAL HYPERPLASIA	EVERY OTHER GENE PATHWAY	DUCTAL (DCIS) ⊕ CALCIFICATIONS	LUMINAL A LUMINAL B HER-2 ENRICHED BASAL LIKE		INVASIVE DUCTAL CARCINOMA	TRIED TO MAKE DUCTLES ⊕ DESMO

Breast Cancer

RISK FACTORS

① MAMMARY GLAND PROLIF
  "CUMULATIVE ESTROGEN"
② TERM PREGNANCY + BREASTFEEDING
  PROGESTIN CYCLES PRL
③ MAMMARY VULNERABLE
  • 1ST TERM < 21   1ST TERM > 35
    ↓½ RISK   ↑ RISK
  • LCIS   MULTIFOCAL, ⑧
  • ANY BAD BX   ↑RISK⑧
  • HRT-ESTROGEN ↓ER⊕
④ AGE GREATEST RISK 1/8 ~75
⑤ BREAST DENSITY, ↑RISK DENSITY
⑥ ANOVULATORY CONTRACEPTION?
  LNG-IUD ⊅HOC NEXPLANON

GENETICS

ALL=PI3KINASE, TP53
BRCA1 = BASAL-LIKE (TP53 1ST)
BRCA2 = LUMINAL B (HIGH-GRADE)
HER2 = HER2-ENRICHED (PROLIF)
LCIS = E-CADHERIN
  ILC CDH1
DCIS = LUMINAL A
  IDC   ER⊕, HER2⊖

SPECIAL TYPES

↳ **LOBULAR (LCIS, ILC)**
PATH: E-CADHERIN, CDH1
  NO DESMOPLASTIC, NO CALCIF
PT: Ø LUMP Ø MAMMO
  NO SCREENING
  INCIDENTAL
BX: LCIS: LOBULAR EXPANSION
ILC: SINGLE, SINGLE - FILE
TX: –

↳ **MAMMARY PAGET'S**
PATH: DCIS INVADE THE
  EPIDERMIS OF NIPPLE
PT: SCALING, ULCERATION
  A ITCHY NIPPLE
  "ECZEMA" FAILS TX
BX: PAGETOID CELLS ⊕
  CK7 ⊕
TX: DCIS, IDC

↳ **INFLAMMATORY CANCER**
PATH: IDC CANCER CELLS
  BUILD DUCTS IN LYMPH
PATH: RED, SWOLLEN, TENDER
  PEAU D'ORANGE
  NIPPLE RETRACTION
BX: DUCTAL CELLS MAKING
  DUCTS IN LYMPH
TX: IDC

DUCTAL TYPES

↳ **LUMINAL A (50%) B (15%)**
PATH: "CLASSIC" DUCTAL
  HIGH GRADE (B), HI KI-67
  BRCA2 CANCER
PT: ASX MAMMOGRAM SCREEN
  OLD WHITE LADY ⊂̄ LUMP
  "↑ ESTROGEN EXPOSURE"
BX: ER⊕ LOW GRADE, HER2⊖
  HIGH-GRADE,↑KI-67
TX: SERM   AROMATASE-I
  (PRE-MEN)   (POST-MEN)

↳ **HER2-ENRICHED (10%)**
PATH: HER2 (RTK, PROMOTES GROWTH)
  PROLIFERATION GENES, ER⁻
PT: SAA, WORSE PROGNOSIS
BX: HER2⁺ ER⁻ ↑KI-67
TX: TRASTUZUMAB

↳ **BASAL-LIKE (15%)**
PATH: BRCA1 GERM-LINE
  TP53 (1ST, NONSENSE)
  ER⁻, PR⁻, HER2⁻
  EGFR (RTK, ØHER2)
PT: YOUNG, YOUNG, YOUNG
  MENARCHE 1ST TERM
  MULTIPOROUS,↓BREASTFEEDING
  BLACK, OBESE
DX: TRIPLE-NEGATIVE
  EGFR⊕ CK56⊕
TX: WORST PROGNOSIS
  NEOADJUVANT

SCREENING U/S

↳ ↑ DETECTION, ↑EARLY TREATMENT, ↓COST
① SBE/CBE = NO   ② U/S ⟹ HARM
③ MAMMORAM GOLD STANDARD
  40 Q/YR OR 50 Q2YR
④ (BRCA1/2) OR (DENSE+↑RISK) MRI
⑤ PPX TAH, BSO, ⑧ MASTECTOMY

SURGICAL TX OF CANCER

① STAGE I AND II
  LUMPECTOMY,   SENTINEL NODE
  RADIATION   OR   DISSECTION
  MASTECTOMY,   SENTINEL NODE
                      DISSECTION
② STAGE III
  MASTECTOMY,   SENTINEL NODE
  CHEMO +/- XRT   DISSECTION
③ STAGE IV
  PALLIATION   –
  RADICAL AXILLARY DISSECTION

CHEMO TO KNOW

① SERM
  TAMOXIFEN = UTERINE CANCER
  RALOXIFENE = DVT
② HEART FAILURE
  TRASTUZUMAB DOSE-INDEPENDENT, REVERSIBLE
  ANTHRACYCLINES CUMULATIVE, IRREVERSIBLE
                   DOSE
③ AROMATASE-I = ADRENAL ANDROGENS
  ANATROZOLE

NOTES

Physiology of Pregnancy

FERROPORTIN DISINHIBITED IN MOM'S GUT AND

OXY BIRTH | ADH ↓SOSM | ??

POST ANT | HYPO

↑ ANT PIT ≥ 2x HYPERPLASIA + HYPERTROPHY LACTOTROPES 3 BV

SHEEHAN'S

CONCURRENT PRL ↑

SPIDER ANGIOMATA

CHORION 6-7 MG/DAY ESTROGEN

HEPCIDIN

PALMAR ERYTHEMA

LIVER

FACTOR 7-10 ↓ PROTEIN C, S
HYPERCOAGUABLE

VESSELS

⊙ AT₁ PROGESTERONE AT₂

ANGZ

ALDO

FETUS CONTRACTIONS

PRELOAD

MARROW

+ RBC + WBC ↑ PLT

PTHRP

PROGESTERONE = SM DILATOR
↳ ↓SVR ↳ ↓GERD ↳ ↓MYOMETRIAL QUIESCENCE
β-HCG = ⊙⊙
↳ MORNING SICKNESS ↳ HYPERTHYROID LAB Δs
↳ HYPEREMESIS GRAVIDARUM ↳ THECA-LUTEIN CYSTS

SUPPLEMENT: CA + VIT D

MOM
↑ 1,25-VIT D
↑ CA, ↑PHOS ABSORPTION
↑ CA, ↑PHOS REABSORPTION
↓ PTH

HGB
10-
12 24 36

PL CATCHES UP

"WATER BREAKING" ROM
↓ CERVICAL DILATION
"BLOODY SHOW"

AMNIOTIC FLUID (FERNING)

MUCUS PLUG (BEADING)

CERVICAL HYPERPLASIA

↑GLYCOPROTEIN ↑LACTOBACILLUS ↑PH

SUPPLEMENTS: Fe + FOLATE

BLOOD PRESSURE

MAP = CO x SVR
        ↑   ↓ PROGESTERONE
   ↑ HR x SV   AT, BLOCKADE
                 (CHORIONIC VILLI)

GRAVITY
LOWER EXT EDEMA
NOCTURIA
ALL FOURS IF ↓BP
⊙ SIDE

CONT x PL
↑ ALDOSTERONE

MAP | VILLI STOP
12 24 36

METABOLISM
INSULIN
HCS

⊖ LIPOLYSIS → FFA → KETONES
NEONATAL LIFE FETUS

POSTPRANDIAL HYPERBG
HYPERINSULINEMIA
PREPRANDIAL HYPOBG

PGH↑⊕

PLACENTA MADE
HCG
% MAX
PGH PROGESTERONE ESTROGEN HCS (hPL)
12 24 36

MOM MADE
% MAX
PROLACTIN
OXYTOCIN
12 24 36

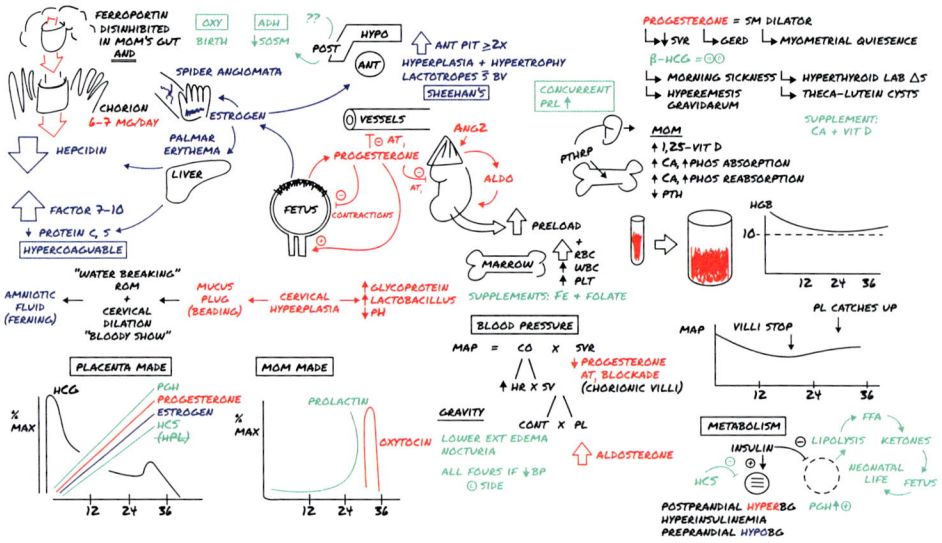

Physiology of Parturition

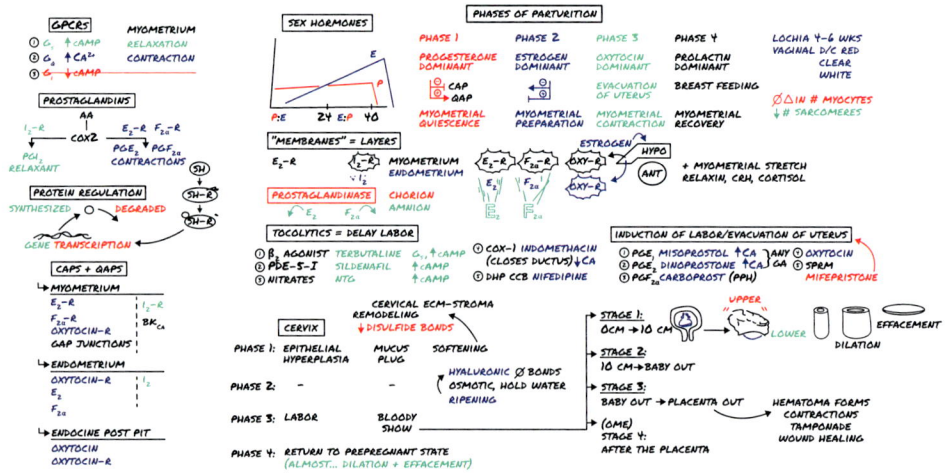

GPCRs | MYOMETRIUM
① Gₛ ↑CAMP | RELAXATION
② Gq ↑CA²⁺ | CONTRACTION
③ Gᵢ ↓CAMP |

SEX HORMONES
E
P
P:E 24 E:P 40

PHASES OF PARTURITION
PHASE 1	PHASE 2	PHASE 3	PHASE 4	LOCHIA 4-6 WKS VAGINAL D/C RED CLEAR WHITE
PROGESTERONE DOMINANT	ESTROGEN DOMINANT	OXYTOCIN DOMINANT	PROLACTIN DOMINANT	
↓ CAP ↓ GAP		EVACUATION OF UTERUS	BREAST FEEDING	
MYOMETRIAL QUIESCENCE	MYOMETRIAL PREPARATION	MYOMETRIAL CONTRACTION	MYOMETRIAL RECOVERY	∅ Δ IN # MYOCYTES ↓ # SARCOMERES

PROSTAGLANDINS
AA
COX2
I₂-R → PGI₂ RELAXANT
E₂-R F₂ₐ-R → PGE₂ PGF₂ₐ CONTRACTIONS

SH
SH-R
SH-R

"MEMBRANES" = LAYERS
E₂-R MYOMETRIUM ENDOMETRIUM I₂
PROSTAGLANDINASE CHORION AMNION
↓E₂ ↓F₂ₐ

E₂-R F₂ₐ-R OXY-R
E₂↑ F₂ₐ↑ OXY-R
E₂↑ F₂ₐ↑

ESTROGEN
HYPO
ANT
+ MYOMETRIAL STRETCH RELAXIN, CRH, CORTISOL

PROTEIN REGULATION
SYNTHESIZED ○ DEGRADED
GENE TRANSCRIPTION

CAPS + GAPS
↳ MYOMETRIUM
E₂-R
F₂ₐ-R
OXYTOCIN-R I₂-R BKCA
GAP JUNCTIONS
↳ ENDOMETRIUM
OXYTOCIN-R I₂
E₂
F₂ₐ
↳ ENDOCINE POST PIT
OXYTOCIN
OXYTOCIN-R

TOCOLYTICS = DELAY LABOR
① β₂ AGONIST TERBUTALINE Gₛ, ↑CAMP
② PDE-5-I SILDENAFIL ↑CAMP
③ NITRATES NTG ↑CAMP

④ COX-1 INDOMETHACIN (CLOSES DUCTUS) ↓CA
⑤ DHP CCB NIFEDIPINE

INDUCTION OF LABOR/EVACUATION OF UTERUS
① PGE₂ MISOPROSTOL ↑CA ANY ⊙ OXYTOCIN
② PGE₂ DINOPROSTONE ↑CA GA ⊙ SPRM
③ PGF₂ₐ CARBOPROST (PPH) MIFEPRISTONE

CERVICAL ECM-STROMA REMODELING
↓ DISULFIDE BONDS

CERVIX
PHASE 1: EPITHELIAL HYPERPLASIA | MUCUS PLUG | SOFTENING
PHASE 2: — — HYALURONIC ∅ BONDS OSMOTIC, HOLD WATER RIPENING
PHASE 3: LABOR | BLOODY SHOW
PHASE 4: RETURN TO PREPREGNANT STATE (ALMOST... DILATION + EFFACEMENT)

STAGE 1: 0CM → 10 CM
UPPER
LOWER
EFFACEMENT
DILATION

STAGE 2: 10 CM → BABY OUT

STAGE 3: BABY OUT → PLACENTA OUT
HEMATOMA FORMS CONTRACTIONS TAMPONADE WOUND HEALING

(OME) STAGE 4: AFTER THE PLACENTA

NOTES

Reproduction

Family Planning and Contraception

	METHOD	HORMONE	DURATION	MECHANISM	NOTES + CHALLENGES
LARC	IMPLANT	ETONOGESTREL	3 YRS	ANOVULATION	CANCER-PREVENTING MENSES-ENDING GET PREGNANT WHEN YOU WANT
	IUD	LEVONORGESTREL / CU-IUD	5 YRS / 10-12 YRS	IMPLANTATION-I + LOCAL EFFECTS IMPLANTATION-I	⬆ BLEEDING NOT
PROGESTIN ONLY	INJECTABLES	MEDROXY-PROGESTERONE	3 MOS	ANOVULATION	WEIGHT GAIN ⬇BMD
	POP		22 HRS	LOCAL EFFECTS	WORST EFFICACY
ESTROGEN + PROGESTIN	VAGINAL RING	ESTRADIOL + PROGESTIN	3 WKS	ANOVULATION	DVT, ≥ 35 YRS + TOBACCO OR ⬆ HYPERCOAGULABLE
	TD PATCH		1 WK		21/7 24/4 84/7
	COC		1 DAY	ESTRADIOL INDUCES PROLIFERATION	HORMONE-FREE INTERVAL IS REQUIRED TO AVOID SPOTTING, CONTROL BLEEDING

HYPO GNRH ANALOGS LEUPROLIDE
↓
ANT PIT
↓
OVULATION COC DHC ETONOGESTREL IMPLANT MEDROXYPROGESTERONE
OVARY
FERTILIZATION BARRIER METHODS Ⓡ TL, VASECTOMY
↓
ENDOMETRIUM IMPLANTATION CU-IUD TAH POP LNG-IUD
PROGESTIN ESTRADIOL NONHORMONAL
ESTROGEN + PROGESTIN

MENSTRUATION = TOLERABLE NUISANCE
↳ EVACUATE UTERUS OF ENDOMETRIUM
↳ PROLIFERATION = MUTATION = CANCER

FAMILY PLANNING
- NOT CONTRACEPTION
- IS PROCONCEPTION
- CHART BASAL TEMP
- CHART CERVICAL MUCUS
- ABSTINENCE FROM SEX
- SEX Ž OVULATION

PERMANENT STERILIZATION
⚥ "VASECTOMY" DUCTUS DEFERENS LIGATED + CUT
♀ BTL HYSTEROSCOPIC TUBAL LIGATION TAH

PRECOITAL (WORST)
♂ MALE CONDOM *STI PREVENTION
♀ FEMALE CONDOM DIAPHRAGM CAPS SPERMICIDE (⬆HIV)

POSTCOITAL, EMERGENCY
PROGESTIN ONLY (LNG) W/I 72 HRS
5PRM W/I 120 HRS
CU-IUD W/I 120 HRS PENNIES?
TYPE TAKE ENOUGH COC TO GET THE PROGESTIN HIGH ENOUGH
+ ESTROGEN TOXICITY = N/V

Pregnancy Pathologies of the Chorion

GTD DISPERMY
= "55" COMPLETE NORMAL
= "59" PARTIAL SPON AB

COMPLETE MOLE
PATH: COMPLETELY MOLAR, CHR #, HYDATID, SPERMAL SYNCYTIO = ⬆ HCG
PT: SIZE-DATE DISCREPANCY HYPEREMESIS GRAVIDARUM HYPERTHYROID, THECA-LUTEIN CYSTS "GRAPE-LIKE" MASS
DX: TVUS = SNOWSTORM, ∅EMBRYO D+C, ∅ BV IN VILLI, ALL HYDROPIC
TX: D+C, RELIABLE CONTRACEPTION NOT IUD
F/U: SERIAL HCG, 6 MO P̄ ∅

PARTIAL (INCOMPLETE) MOLE
PATH: OPPOSITE OF ABOVE CYTOTROPHOBLAST = ∅ HCG
PT: NORMAL PREGNANCY UNTIL U/S
DX: TVUS = SNOWSTORM, ⊕EMBRYO D+C, ∅BV IN VILLI, SOME VILLI
TX: SAA
F/U: SAA
COMPLETE →ᵐ GTN, ⊕ CHORIO
PARTIAL →ᵐ GTN, ∅ CHORIO

GTN INVASIVE MOLE
PREGNANCY CHORIO-CARCINOMA
EPITHELIOID PSTT
"GTN"
PATH: NO VILLI, METASTATIC: CHORIO @VILLI, LOCAL: INVASIVE
PT: SERIAL HCG DID NOT REACH ∅, PLATEAUED, OR RISE AND ASX ON CONTRACEPTION
DX: STAGING CT TVUS, BX, D+C
TX: METHOTREXATE (ACTINOMYCIN-D)
F/U: SERIAL HCG, 12 MO P̄ ∅

FIGO
- AGE
- # ORGANS (LUNGS 1ˢᵗ)
- TYPE OF PREGNANCY
- TIMING OF PREGNANCY
- HCG @ DIAGNOSIS

PERCRETA
INCRETA   ACCRETA

IMPLANTATION INTO SCARRED ENDO
MULTIPAROUS, SURGICAL UTERUS
"PREVIA"
PATH: IMPLANTATION OVER CERVICAL OS OS DILATES = VESSELS TEAR PLACENTAL MIGRATION "PANCAKE SEDUCTION" BABY BLEEDS
PT: PAINLESS VAGINAL BLEEDING Ž CERVICAL DILATION, ONSET OF LABOR OR
ASX SCREENING U/S
TX: CESAREAN SECTION
PLACENTA PREVIA
VASA PREVIA
"ACCRETA"
PATH: IMPLANTATION IS TOO DEEP NO ENDOMETRIUM = ∅ SHEDDING IF DELIVERED = MOM BLEEDS
PT: PAINLESS VAGINAL BLEEDING Ž DELIVERY OF PLACENTA, END OF LABOR OR
ASX SCREENING TVUS
DX: TVUS
TX: PERIPARTUM TAH Ž ELECTIVE CESAREAN
F/U: DELIVER = HEMORRHAGE LEAVE IT = ENDOMETRITIS

LATE COMPLICATIONS
↳ PLACENTAL ABRUPTION
PATH: SEPARATION Ž CONTRACTIONS MOM BLEEDS
PT: PAINFUL VAGINAL BLEEDING BEFORE ONSET OF LABOR AND DECELERATION, ⬇BP (COCAINE)
DX: TVUS
TX: CESAREAN
CONCEALED
UTERINE RUPTURE
PATH: MYOMETRIAL CONTRACTIONS RIP OPEN SCAR, DELIVERY INTO PELVIS
CRASH   ELECTIVE   SCAR DOESN'T CONTRACT
PT: PAINFUL ⬆S, +/- VAG BLEEDING DURING LABOR, LOSS OF FETAL STATION, ⬇UTERUS
DX: CLX
TX: CRASH SECTION
F/U: VBAC TOLAC

© 2021 OnlineMedEd

NOTES

Pregnancy Pathologies of the Amnion

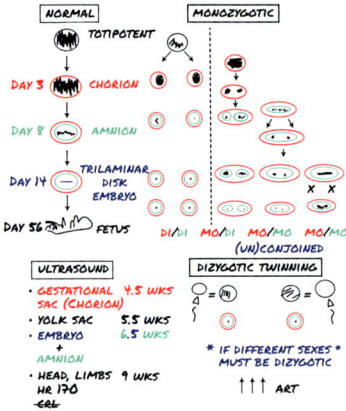

NORMAL
- TOTIPOTENT
- DAY 3 — CHORION
- DAY 8 — AMNION
- DAY 14 — TRILAMINAR DISK / EMBRYO
- DAY 56 — FETUS

MONOZYGOTIC

DI/DI   MO/DI   MO/MO   MO/MO
(UN)CONJOINED

ULTRASOUND
- GESTATIONAL SAC (CHORION) 4.5 WKS
- YOLK SAC 5.5 WKS
- EMBRYO + AMNION 6.5 WKS
- HEAD, LIMBS 9 WKS
- HR 170
- CRL

DIZYGOTIC TWINNING

* IF DIFFERENT SEXES * MUST BE DIZYGOTIC

↑↑↑ ART

ECTOPIC PREGNANCY

PATH: IMPLANTATION, NOT UTERUS 90% TUBAL, 70% AMPULLA IMPAIRED PASSAGE (SCAR)

PT: **PRE-RUPTURE:** PREGNANCY MISSED MENSES, ⊕ UPT VAGINAL SPOTTING, ABD PAIN
POST-RUPTURE: PERITONITIS HEMOPERITONEUM, HGB INSPIRATION = SHOULDER PAIN

DX: TVUS, β-HCG
TX: SMALL: MTX ± F/U
SICK: SALPINGECTOMY
ØSICK: SALPINGOSTOMY
F/U: EQUAL RATE OF RECURRENCE DESIRED FUTURE FERTILITY

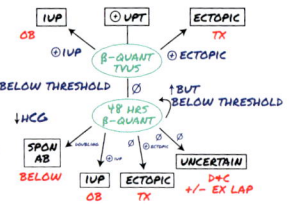

IUP — OB   ⊕ UPT   ECTOPIC — TX
⊕ IUP   β-QUANT TVUS   ⊕ ECTOPIC
BELOW THRESHOLD   Ø   ↑ BUT BELOW THRESHOLD
↓ HCG   48 HRS β-QUANT
SPON AB   Ø
BELOW   IUP — OB   ECTOPIC — TX   UNCERTAIN   D+C +/- EX LAP

SPONTANEOUS ABORTION = MISCARRIAGE, FETAL DEMISE, FETAL LOSS

TYPE	PASSAGE OF CONTENTS	CERVICAL OS	U/S	NOTES
IUP	Ø	CLOSED	ALIVE	OB CARE
THREATENED	Ø	CLOSED	ALIVE	IS VAGINAL BLEEDING
INEVITABLE	Ø	OPEN	DEAD	PPROM PREVIABLE GESTATION
INCOMPLETE	⊕	OPEN	RETAINED PARTS	SURGERY > MEDICAL > EXPECTANT
COMPLETE	⊕	CLOSED	EMPTY	RHO(D) STATUS
MISSED	Ø	CLOSED	DEAD	SURGERY > MEDICAL > EXPECTANT

BABY IS ALREADY DEAD

SURGICAL
SUCTION D+C = 1ST TRI
SUCTION D+C = 2ND TRI

CERVICAL RIPENING
HYDROSCOPIC DILATORS
MISOPROSTAL

MEDICALLY
MIFEPRISTONE (SPRM)
MISOPROSTAL (PGE₁)
METHOTREXATE
DINOPRISTONE (PGE₂)
OXYTOCIN (OXY)

40- / 36- VIABLE
24- / 20- PRE VIABLE
0- NON VIABLE

194

© 2021 OnlineMedEd

NOTES